HOW TO LEARN
MUSCLE CONTROL

BY
OTTO ARCO AND ALAN CALVERT

Originally Published in 1925

PUBLISHED BY O'Faolain Patriot LLC,
Copyright 2012 info@PhysicalCultureBooks.com

Published in the United States of America

ISBN-13: 978-1477633137

ISBN-10: 1477633138

To Order More Copies Visit: Physical Culture
Books.com

The information contained in this publication is for historical and educational purposes only and is not designed to and does not provide medical, nutritional, or health advice, diagnosis, or opinion for any health or individual problem. The material presented is not a substitute for medical or other professional health services from a qualified health care provider who is familiar with the unique facts of the individual, and should not be used in place of a visit, call, consultation, or advice of a physician or other healthcare provider. Individuals should always consult a qualified health care provider about any health concern and prior to undertaking any new treatment. The publisher assumes no responsibility and specifically disclaims all liability for any consequence relating directly or indirectly to any action or inaction that a reader takes based on any information contained herein.

Be advised that no one should undertake exercises in the nature of those addressed in this book without prior consultation with a physician. Nor does the publisher make any representation concerning whether any of the exercises or suggestions provided by the trainers or physical fitness specialists featured in this book would be effective or appropriate for the reader's needs or expectations. The publisher expressly disclaims any and all responsibility and/or liabilities that might result from the uninformed or misinformed application of the techniques identified herein as

How to Learn Muscle Control

THIS article, which is the first of a series, is the joint work of Otto Arco and myself. The division of labor is somewhat unequal. Arco does all the work of posing and supplies all the details of instruction. All that I do is to get the material together, to expand his all-too-brief notes, to comment on his ideas and attend to the publication.

Personally I have been familiar with the subject of muscle-control since thirty years ago, when I saw it demonstrated by Checkley, by Sandow and by the dozens of performers who imitated his posing act.

Sandow used muscle-control as a part of his posing; that is, many of his poses depended for their effectiveness on his ability to control, and thus display, his muscles. Those who reproduced his act, reproduced his poses, as well as they could; but there was no decided advance in the art of muscle-control until Arco came along.

He not only was able to duplicate all the control feats of his predecessor, but by reason of his study and knowledge, could and did, originate a lot of new feats; getting his own muscles under the control of his will to a degree that no one else has been able to even approximate—much less equal.

He taught much of what he knew to some of his personal friends and fellow artists, and there have been courses issued by others, courses based on information received from Arco. Which bothered him not at all. "For," as he says, "muscle control is a good thing for anyone to have. If I have helped these other fellows to teach it, I feel I have done both them and the public a good turn."

Since he has lived in the country he has been a perfect mine of information to those enthusiasts who are interested in the subject. Time and again, he has given up his time to answering letters begging for instruction on matters of detail; and has done so out of the kindness of his heart.

In that connection I must here say that Arco is an extremely busy man, with but little time for letter-writing. A set of articles like this is sure to give some of you the idea of writing for personal advice. At present it is impossible for either of us to give personal instruction, but if any of you think that he must write to Arco, then please address your letter to him in care of this magazine. If your letter raises a question of general interest—something which if answered would help other enthusiasts—it will be probably answered in these pages. If on the other hand the question is entirely personal, the letter may not be answered, Arco is working on this series at a considerable sacrifice of his own time and convenience: so let's not make it hard for him by asking him for purely personal service.

Shortly after this series was announced, Arco had to leave for an extended tour of the Orpheum Circuit; so some of you who live in the west have had the opportunity to see his act; and you probably noticed that his posing, his series of muscle control stunts, interested the audience even more than did his remarkable acrobatic feats.

His ability to make his muscles perform, his ability to control them, is positively weird; and seemingly his audiences are fascinated by his ability in that line.

He writes me that whenever he plays a return engagement at a theatre, the manager is almost sure to ask him to alter his act, so as to give more posing.

So he knows that people like his posing. He realizes that many who follow out these instructions will do so for the purpose of becoming able to amaze others by demonstrations of almost unbelievable control of the muscles.

But he contends that posing is merely a side issue. The main purpose of muscle-control is self-mastery. Muscle control involves far more than the mere ability to make the muscles contract. It teaches you to relax, which is sometimes even more important than contraction. It gives you a selective control, and therefore the ability to single out those muscles necessary to the work to be done, and only those muscles; leaving the antagonistic, or non-helpful, muscles relaxed. That makes a saving of energy in two ways; since it enables you to put all your energy into stimulating the needed muscles, and relieves those muscles of the interference of needlessly flexed antagonistic muscles.

Muscle control, which leads to body-control, is a great factor for success in all competitive sports. Your ability to shine in any outdoor game rests in your ability to make your body do exactly what you want it to do. Bodily control is the secret of that skill which is dependent on co-ordination and timing. As an illustration. Consider the style of a champion golfer as compared to a beginner. The expert makes his shot with perfect smoothness and rhythm, getting great distance and extreme accuracy, without any noticeable muscular exertion. He has his arms and body so thoroughly under control that he can perform any shot needed. The novice holds himself nervously tense, uses only his arms instead of employing a body swing, and gets nowhere. Only by repeated practice can he will his body so that it will respond to the commands of his will. Any golf instructor will tell you that there are some beginners who seem to be utterly lacking in body control. They cannot make their bodies behave, cannot carry out a single command; such as shifting the weight from one foot to another, executing a body swing, or a follow through; and even cannot imitate movements made by the instructor. Such men lack that bodily mastery which depends on muscle control.

It would be possible to go in and give several instances of the importance of bodily control in other sports, tennis, baseball, billiards, rowing, etc.

But Arco claims that the benefit that comes from learning muscle control is not limited to its application to athletics. He says that it is even more helpfulness to the nervous system than to the muscles; because as each muscular contraction is the result of a nerve message your practice brings the nerves under control not only gives you the power to stimulate the muscles to greater effect, but also enables you to relax, at will, both the nerves and muscles.

Anything which increases the domination of the mind over the body is a good thing. And anything which gives one "nerve" and cures "nerves" is likewise a good thing. You can use this muscle-control as a basis of acquiring will-control and nerve-control. If you happen to be a baseball pitcher you cannot only get that kind of muscle and body control which enables you to throw a ball how and where you want it to go; but you can further acquire that self-control which enables you to pitch perfectly in unfavorable conditions and before a hostile crowd.

Arco claims that learning muscle control will enable you to control your temper, to control your habits and, through strengthening your will power, to control your morals. That sounds like a large order, as though he was claiming too much; but the fact remains that will-power can be developed just the same way that a muscle can; vis. by intelligent use.

Neither Arco nor I claim that this practice of muscle-control will make the muscles very much bigger. But it will make them stronger by making them more alive, more responsive to the will, and it will alter and improve their shape because certain of the stunts can be performed only by the ultimate contraction of some muscles; and those muscles have to be gradually educated up to the point where they can make these extreme contractions.

There are other benefits which can be mentioned. This first article deals entirely with control of the upper back muscles, but where you come later on to the studies of abdominal control you will find that they will be of a great advantage to your digestive organs: the practice of the stunts affording the organs a sort of natural massage which does for them just what the rational exercise does for the muscles.

Personally I recommend all these muscle control stunts because they will help you in acquiring posture and balance and that absolute correctness of muscular co-ordination which does so much to promote the automatic growth of muscular tissue.

When I have trouble in teaching posture, it is because the man I am talking to is utterly unable to control the separate parts of his body. If I tell him to throw out his chest, he pulls back his shoulders; having no ability to move the chest independently of the shoulders. When I tell him to lift the front of the hips, he does just the opposite; and if I tell him to try and straighten the lower half of his spine, he is as helpless to obey as if I had asked him to do some difficult contortion stunt. I know that this muscle control will help in that respect.

INSTRUCTIONS

Before you can control your muscles, the first thing to learn is relaxation. When giving instruction in piano playing Padarewski will use the word "relax" dozens of times in one lesson. It is impossible to teach any set of muscles to contract in a certain way, to do something new, if the proper action of these muscles is limited and hampered by the contraction (tension) of other neighboring muscles.

So, you will find at the start that some of those stunts are impossible of performance unless you start off by relaxing; and that when Arco says to relax certain muscles he means it.

Take for a start the control of the shoulder blades, or lo he accurate of the muscles which move the shoulder blades. It is a curious co-incidence that I should have written that editorial about the collar bones just before I started to prepare this article, look at the pictures. That exercise is really a muscle-control stunt; and for the shoulder blades. It is a simple elementary movement, which nevertheless, some of you will find it difficult to do at your first attempt. Now read on and see how much more completely and effectually Arco teaches you this control of the shoulder blades. He says, first, to sit in an arm-chair with your elbows resting on the chair-arms, and all your muscles relaxed. Now try and shrug your shoulders. In an ordinary shrug you would raise your shoulders towards your ears; but if you keep your arm muscles relaxed and your elbows against the arms of the chair, why! then your shoulders cannot rise. But the effort to "shrug" will result in a slight lifting of the shoulder-blades. You can feel them moving under the skin; feel them moving away from the ribs. With each day's practice you will gain extra control, become able to move the blades more and more independently of the rest of the body; and the blades instead of being muscle-bound, as before, will become looser; and you will have consequently more "play", more range of movement in the shoulders themselves.

The next step is to learn to do the same thing with the arms held out straight to the sides. Keep your arms still, with their muscles relaxed, and shrug the shoulders. You can easily tell whether you are successful by the feel of the shoulder-blades moving; crawling as it were up and down the back.

Then stand in front of your mirror with arms outstretched, and body completely relaxed. Jam your shoulder-blades together until they touch; then spread them as you would if you wanted to reach the furthest distance possible to the sides.

Next try to do the shrug as you spread the blades (as in Figure I) ; and relax the dorsal muscles (letting the shoulders drop) as you "jam": and you will find that the shoulder-blades have been curling outwards.

Next—relax the back muscles when spreading; and shrug as you jam the shoulder-blades together, as in Figure II; and your shoulder-blades will circle inwards.

A good way of learning these movements is to stand with your back to a wall opposite the mirror; with your arms outstretched, and try to describe circles with your shoulders. Not with your hands, mind you; for the arms are always horizontal and relaxed; but the points of the shoulders should describe circles. Therefore watch not the arms but the shoulders. Don't be discouraged, if at first the movement is small. It is bound to be small in the case of every beginner, but the more you learn to control the blades, the more "play" there will be in the shoulders; and the more spectacular will be the movement.

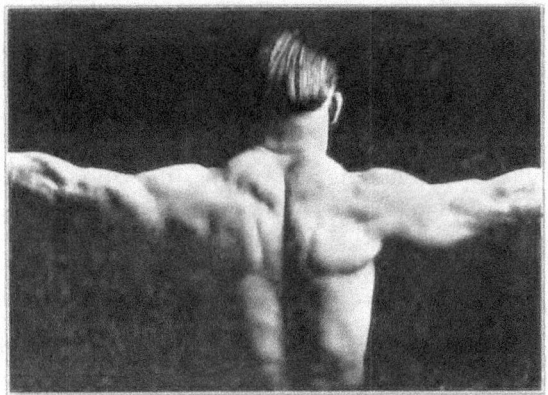

Plate I

The next exercise is the same, but instead of holding the arms out straight, as in Figures I and II, you bend them at the elbows as in Figures III and IV. If you do it this way, you somehow get the latissimus dorsi muscles spread further out to the sides. I can make myself two inches wider across the back when I bend the elbows than when I hold the arms straight. ("I think I must have raised my shoulders, instead of spreading them, when posing for these two pictures as I should have looked much wider than I do."—Arco.) In the four preceding stunts it is very important to keep the arm muscles and trapezius muscles relaxed at all

13

times as that allows you to get the control of the back muscles which move the shoulder-blades.

Before attempting the next three stunts you should make a small ring of rope, or heavy cord, the ring to be about three inches in diameter. Slip the fingers in the ring, raise the arms straight above the head, reaching as high as possible), relax the shoulder muscles, keep the arms rigid, and then pull hard against the rope ring, as though you were trying to break it by moving the hands sideways and away from each other. Particular care should be taken not to bend the arms at the elbows.

If you do this while standing in front of a mirror, and if you will follow the directions properly, you will notice that the sides bulge a little bit, just below the level of the arm-pits. With each day's practice the bulge will become greater until finally the projections caused by the movement of the shoulder blades will appear as half circles as shown in Figures V, VI and VII

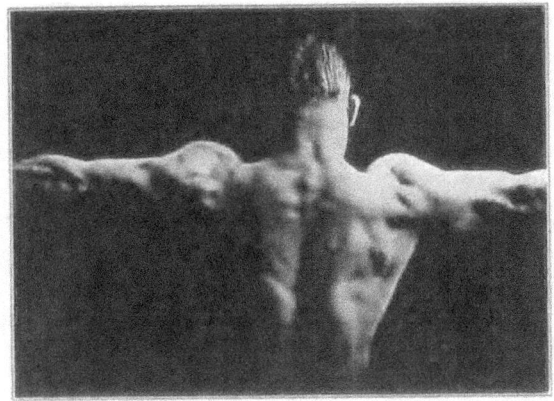

FIGURE II

Supposing that you had your hands aloft as in Figure VII, without holding the rope ring or interlacing your fingers. When you brought the arms sideways and downwards, the motive power would be supplied by the muscles on the upper back, which are attached to the upper arm bones, and which by their contraction bring the arms down. But when you do hold the rope-ring and pull vigorously against it, those back muscles contract: and because the arms are held together with the rope ring the effect is to lift the shoulder-blades apart.

When you first try it all your efforts should be devoted to pulling hard against the rope ring. As the practice continues, and the movement of the shoulder-blades becomes greater you should lessen the pull with the hands and concentrate on projecting the shoulder-blades to the sides.

After you have had fair success with No. VII, try the same thing with the hands on top of the head as in Figures V and VI. When the arms are bent in this way it is more difficult to spread the shoulder-blades, and so this stunt is possible only after you have thoroughly mastered the stunt shown in Figure VII. In Figure VI you can just barely see the rope-ring to which Arco is holding. Of course he can do this stunt without either holding on to a ring, or even clasping the hands: because he has his shoulder-blades under perfect control of his will. In conclusion, you must remember that you will not be able to accomplish either of the stunts shown in Figure V or VII unless you raise the shoulders as high as possible before you start to force the shoulder-blades apart. Also bear in mind that your control of the shoulder-blades is just as much dependent on your ability to relax some of the muscles, as it is on your ability to contract other muscles.

The odd effect in Figures V, VI and VII is due to the fact that the lower points of the shoulder blades have moved upward and outward.

Now, when the blades are in a normal position, they are maintained in that position by the combined action of several muscles. To make the lower points of the blades travel outward to the side, as in Figure VII, you have to contract the muscles which pull the points outwards, while relaxing the opposing muscles, which, if contracted would pull the lower part of the blades inward and towards the spine.

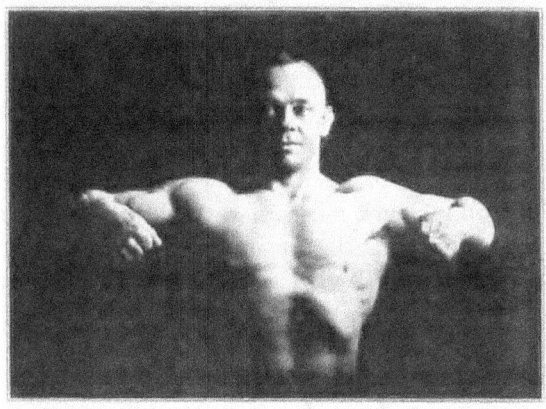

Figure III

That sounds rather complicated but it is something which you must understand before you can make any great progress in these, or in the following stunts of muscle control. In the present case, if you flexed all the muscles attached to the shoulder-blades, and flexed them all with equal vigor, then the blade would remain immovable. But by flexing one set of muscles and relaxing its opposing set you can make the shoulder-blades move in almost any direction you wish.

Arco says that if you can master shoulder-blade control in continual practice, the very fact that you have subjected the upper back muscles to the control of the will, will make it easier for you to yet a mental domination over the other muscles.

In learning to control the shoulder-blades in the four previous stunts you obtained a certain measure of control of the trapezius muscle; since in one or two of those movements the trapezius had to be contracted, and in the others had to be relaxed. Never forget that the word control means ability to relax the muscles at will, just as much as to contract them. The purpose of the stunts shown in Figures I to VII was first, to enable you to move the shoulder-blades to and from each other (spread and jam) and second, to move the lower points of the blades outward and upwards. The purpose of the next two stunts is to give you the power to control the trapezius and some of the other muscles attached to the shoulder blades, so that you will be able to move the other muscles of the blades away from the spine.

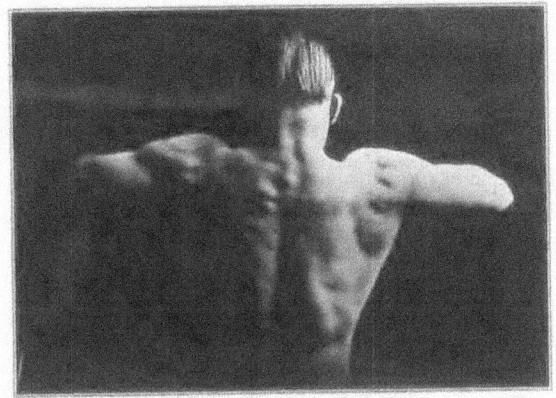

Figure IV

Start out by gripping the rope-ring above your head as in Figure V; relax the shoulders and the back muscles completely. Keep pulling hard against the cord ring and slowly lower your outstretched arms to the front (in a half-circle movement) until the hands are in front of the abdomen as in Figure VIII. (Arco has discarded the ring and is pulling on his left wrist with his right hand.) As your arms come down you will feel the inner edges of the shoulder-blades—the edges nearest the spine—pushing outwards against the skin. Then if you tilt your head back, the trapezius muscles will contract and stick out in those two huge lumps shown in Figures VIII and IX between the sides of the neck and the points of the shoulders.

The last stunt in this lesson is the one shown in Figure X. Rest the back of the hands against the lower part of the spine, and then press as hard against your neck with the back of the hands as you possibly can. At the same time raise your head up and tilt it back. This will make the inner edges of the shoulder-blades project slightly; and with practice you will finally be able to make them stick out as far as Arco's are in the picture.

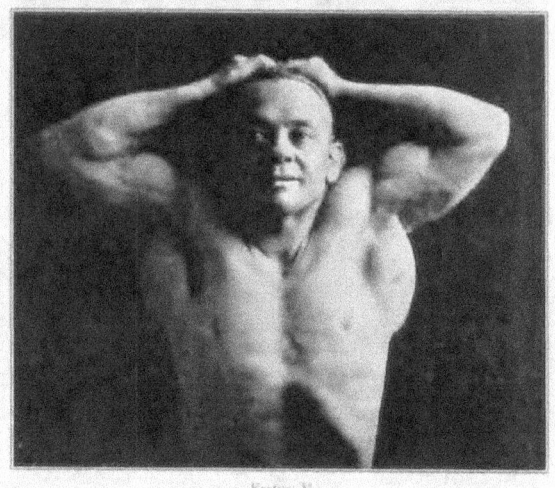

Fictum V

I am fully aware that when some of our readers first see the accompanying pictures they may think that it would be foolish to put in a lot of time practicing for the sake of being able to distort their bodies into such positions. These pictures are spectacular but to some they will seem unsightly. So I wish to repeat that the main object of the training is not the poses themselves, but the muscle control which makes those poses possible. In other words the poses are not the end, but the means of training - of bringing all the body under the domination of your will.

As stated in the first part of this article both Mr. Arco and I are willing to answer questions in the pages of this magazine. I prepared this article under difficulties. Arco is a couple of thousand miles away, whereas he should have been sitting right along side of me to help me with his advice. When I requested him to pose for the pictures I suggested that in each pose he would flex only the muscles necessary to the performance of each stunt and he should deliberately relax all the other muscles of the body. He highly approved of this idea and carried it out except in one or two instances, when he obviously forgot himself. You see it is this way. When Arco is posing on the stage he always makes his body look its very best. Even if he is doing a stunt of abdominal control he will flex the muscles of his arms, shoulders, and legs so as to get a good general effect. It has become sort of a habit with him. But in pictures V, and VI he has flexed only the upper back muscles. I have other pictures showing him in this same pose where his shoulder blades project just as much, and where his upper arms look very much bigger and where the chest and abdomen are strongly flexed. Those pictures are much more wonderful than Figures V and VI. both because they show this power of simultaneous control over all his muscles, and because his arms and the front half of his body are so impressive. So don't judge from the way Arco looks by those pictures V and VI. In them he is deliberately letting his arms relax to show you how you should let your arms relax.

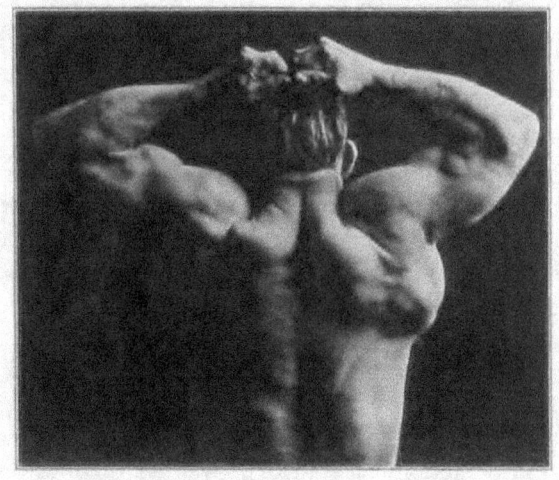

FIGURE VI

If you will refer back, you will see that Arco said that in doing the stunts shown in I and II all the muscles should be relaxed. The next time I see him I am going to ask him to explain why it is that the upper anus and deltoid muscles are relaxed in Figure I and why they are so strongly flexed in Figure II. Whether the act of spreading the shoulder apart caused a contraction of the triceps and deltoids, or whether he forgot himself and flexed those muscles in doing pose II? The difference is very apparent in the two pictures. In I the right triceps is relaxed and hanging of its own weight. In II it is strongly contracted and the upper arm looks very much bigger than it does in Figure I.

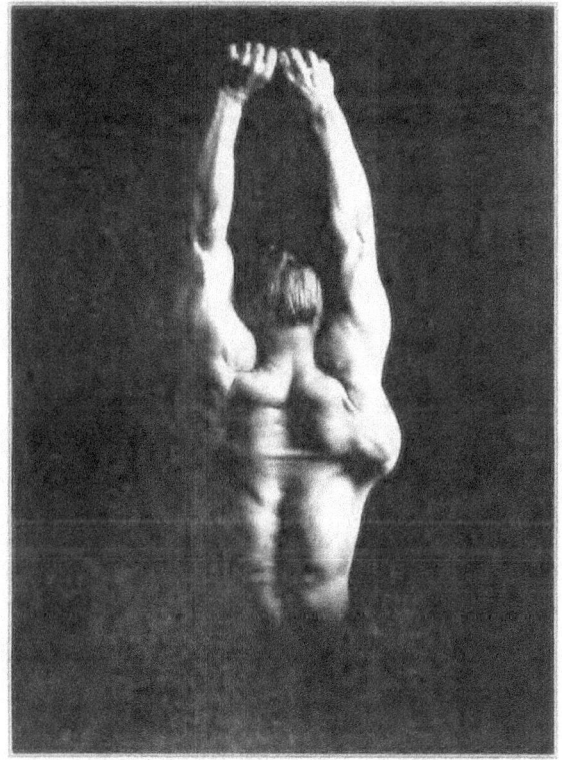

Figure VII

You have thirty days in which to practice this group of stunts, but even in that length of time you can make considerable progress, if you devote a few minutes daily to practice. The difference between muscle control and other forms of exercise is that muscular control does not produce any exhaustion: though it may cause local soreness. In fact Arco says that to master the pose shown in Figure VII may cause considerable pain and that the more pain you can stand the quicker progress you will make.

He calls V, VI and VII dislocation stunts. There is no actual dislocation as far as I can see, except that the top edges of the latissimus muscle overlap the lower points of the shoulder-blades. When you do the stunt VII you actually pull the point of the shoulder-blade from under the edge of the latissimus: which might, I suppose, be called a dislocation. You might think it would be hard to get the points of the blades back again where they belong; that is under the top edge of the latissimus: but they seem to slip back naturally into place. You need not be afraid of any permanent dislocation; for as you gain the ability to move the blades out of place you gain an equal ability to replace them.

In writing the foregoing I have attempted to convey to you as accurately as possible the instructions given in Arco's notes.

I frankly confess that there were one or two points which were obscure to me, and on which I put my own interpretation. For example, he in more than one place says "relax the dorsal muscles." Since a dorsal muscle is a back muscle—that is any back muscle—I have assumed that he meant the latissimus dorsi muscles. But an explanation of this detail will be included in the next issue.

Also I notice that Arco uses the word "shrug" in a different sense from what I would use it. If you, or I, were to shrug our shoulders we would lift the points of the shoulders two or three inches: until they were level with the bottom of our ears. But Arco himself does not shrug his shoulders that way: a fact I have often noticed, since has the habit of "shrugging" as a substitute for saying unpleasant things. (If he is told that someone is stealing his act. or is claiming credit for something he did; or if he is asked a question to which his answer would discredit someone else, he neither protests in the first instance, nor does he reply in the second, but dismisses the disagreeable subject with a philosophical shrug of the shoulders.) And when he shrugs he lifts the points of his shoulders very little, but sort of hunches up the shoulders and neck very much as in Figure VIII. So the question arises whether in the first stunt (Figures I and II) when he says "shrug" he means to lift the points of the shoulders (as he seems to have done in Figure I) or whether he wants you to shrug as he does: by a contraction of the trapezius muscles. I advise you however to lift the shoulders as you will find it much easier to get the rotation of the shoulder blades, than if you were to shrug by a contraction of the trapezius muscle.

This set of muscle-control stunts will be of great help to any man who is troubled by projecting shoulder-blades. There are quite a number of people whose shoulder-blades project at all times: not as much as in Figure X, perhaps, but still there will be a distinct ridge on either side of the spine, caused by the outward pressure on the inner edges of the shoulder-blades. I have been consulted in many such cases, and I could tell that some of those who wrote to me actually thought that they were deformed; whereas the cause of the trouble was nothing more than a bad muscular habit. There are some physical culturists who evidently think that a large neck is a sign of strength, and in order to make the neck appear large they "hunch" the shoulders. That is bound to make the shoulder blades project.

The cure is to relax the trapezius muscles, and, after that is done, the blades will immediately fall into their normal position; and the upper back will be flat and shapely, instead of being deformed with the two projecting ridges. So, any of you that suffer from that disfigurement can remedy it by learning to relax. You will notice that Arco places a great deal of emphasis on this power of voluntary relaxation.

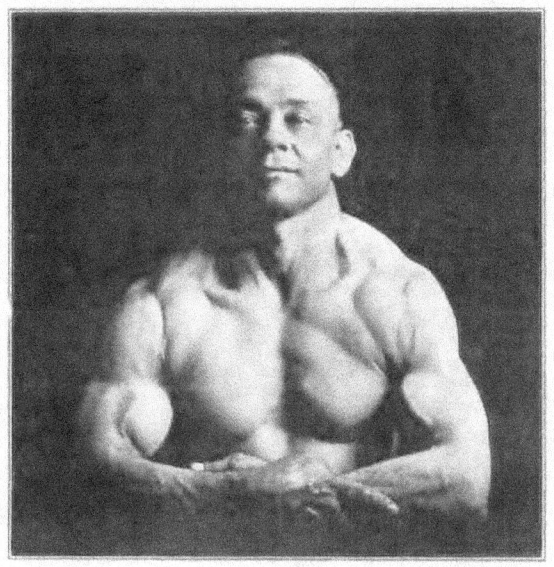

Figure VIII

As I write I have before me a letter written by a gentleman in Chicago, he reports that he had a long interview with Arco and that in discussing muscle control Arco said "that any man could contract his muscles, but that only the expert could relax them."

If you find it easy to master the stunts of shoulder-blade control shown in Figures I to VII, you can if you wish try the one shown in Figure XI. It will be a good test of your ability to contract some muscles while purposely relaxing others. Arco says this stunt is done by holding one arm and shoulder rigid, and pulling vigorously with the other arm.

For example if you want only the right shoulder blade to project you keep the left arm rigid and pull vigorously against the rope ring with the right arm. This is a much harder stunt than the one shown in Figure VII, because it requires you to think of several things at the same time.

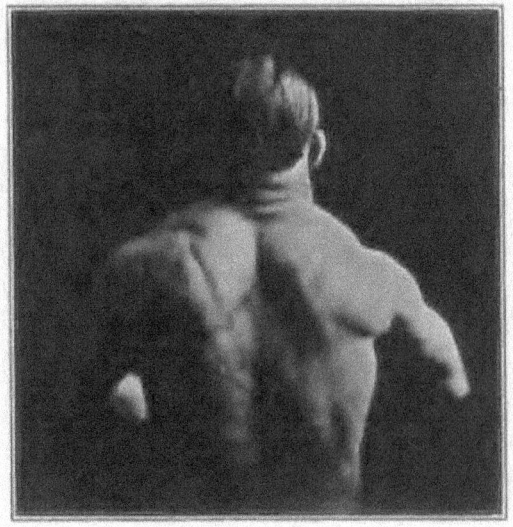

Figure IX

Some of you will undoubtedly wonder why it is that in one part of the magazine I advocate posture and habit as the best body developers and muscle developers and in this muscle control section apparently reverse myself, and recommend exercises which are to be performed every day. All I can say is that these muscle-control stunts are not so much exercises, as studies. The purpose in doing them is not just to exercise the muscles, but to educate them—to increase their power to either contract or relax at the dictate of your will. I know men who have used Indian Clubs and light dumbbells for a half-hour every day over a period of years, and yet after all their training are not able to do even the simplest stunts of muscle-control. On the other hand I have never known a man to lose the power of controlling his muscles once he has mastered it.

You will find some of these stunts very hard to learn, but if you do master them you will never lose the ability to make them perform.

A man whose muscles are already large and powerful will find it easier to acquire the art of muscle control, than will a man whose muscles have never been exercised. The trained gymnast, or the accomplished athlete, whose success is due to his ability to use his muscles will master muscle control stunts with comparatively little trouble. But the man who lets his muscles become lax through neglect of exercise, or by allowing his body to sag, will find it hard to master the stunts. The last named men are exactly the ones who most need to learn muscle control. All exercise involves alternate relaxation and contraction of the muscles. In learning these muscle control stunts you get that muscular contraction and relaxation without the exhaustion attendant on the performance of calisthenic movements, bending exercises, or the more violent forms of sport and athletics.

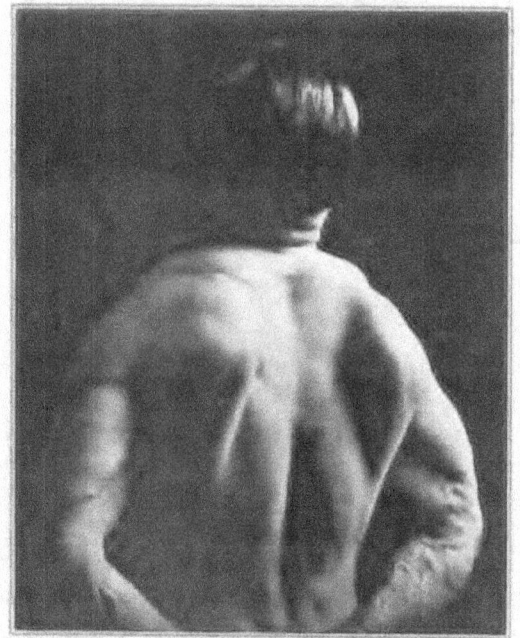

Figure X

After a man has mastered the art of complete muscle control, he can get all necessary exercise by rehearsing the different stunts: and furthermore he can do the stunts wherever he is or however he happens to be costumed.

When he first toured America, it was noted that Sandow did practically no training, and apparently took no exercise whatever outside of the work he got in his vaudeville act. When asked how he exercised he replied that he could get all the exercise he needed to keep himself in perfect shape and condition just by flicking the muscles. He frequently took that kind of exercise during the fifteen minutes he devoted to reading the morning newspaper. In other words he did muscle control stunts. Like Arco, Sandow was such an expert at muscle control that he could do most of the smuts without the necessity of putting his arms into any special position or by using any artificial aids, such as a rope-ring. As you progress you will gain a like ability. For instance you would be able to do the stunts shown in Figure VIII without having to first raise the arms above the head and lower them. You will have gained such control you will be able to flex the trapezius muscles and project the shoulder-blades with the hands folded loosely in the lap. In fact you will be able to flex and relax every muscle on your body and limbs without any noticeable alteration in your position.

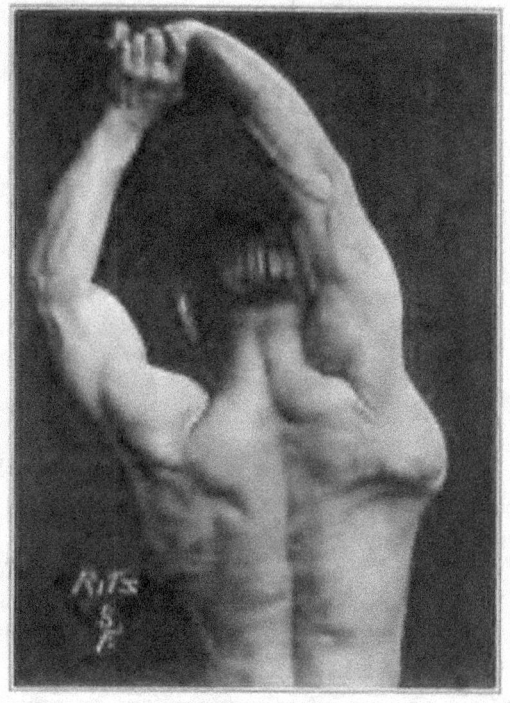

FIGURE XI

Arco wished me to tell you that he is deliberately
holding back some of the information necessary to
absolute control. He said that when it came to the
last lesson in the series he was going to tell you
something— some particular secret of his own—
which would enable you to augment your control
by 50 percent to 100 per cent. Accordingly, I asked
him why he would not give me that information in
the first lesson: to which he replied that to give the

information at the start would only confuse and distract the pupils. He said "it is like this. No one can be a great piano player unless he plays with expression. Just the same, it would be a great mistake to try and teach musical interpretation to a beginner at the piano. First of all, he must learn the notes, and how to use his lingers. He must get his technique, and control of the key-board before he is ready to interpret music. If you tried to teach him to play with expression before he learnt his scales and chords you would distract him. It is just as hard to learn the technique of muscle-control as to learn the technique of piano playing. These readers of yours must first learn the positions favorable to control, and acquire the power of contraction and relaxation. In doing that they will become good at muscular control. After they have learnt to do all these stunts I will tell them some secrets which will make them great at muscular control."

What these secrets are I cannot tell you. I think that Arco is wise not to tell them even to me. I might forget myself and pass them on to you without realizing that I was doing it.

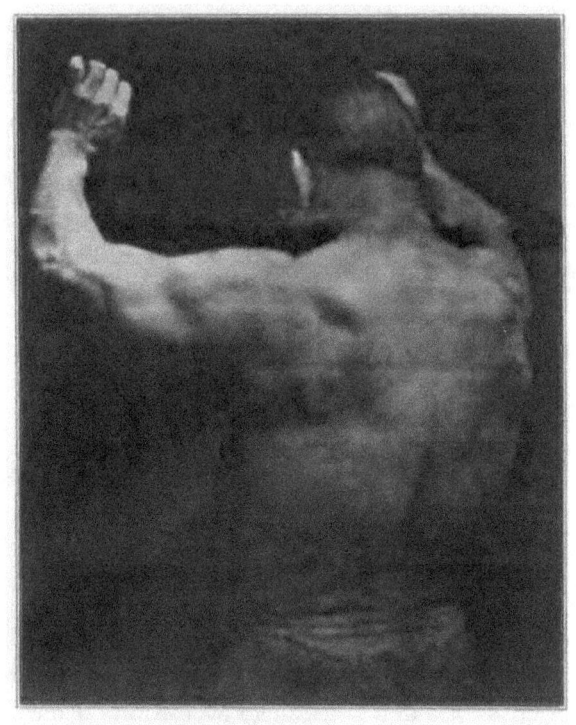

Otto Arco

A good picture with which to finish the article. It shows his ability to relax the muscles on the upper back, while flexing and displaying the great latissimus dorsi muscles; which cover the broad of the back from arm-pit to waist line.

SECOND LESSON

LET us start by assuming that you have practiced the stunts shown in Figures I to IV in the August issue; that you have advanced so far that you can move the shoulder- blades up or down, or towards or away from the spine, when you have your arms raised out to the side. Perhaps you have gone even further, and can move the shoulders in side-wise circles, as suggested by Arco.

If so, you have made a start, but only a start. To contract a muscle (and thereby move some part of the body) is comparatively easy when you place the body or limbs in a position favorable to that contraction. It becomes difficult when you attempt to make the contraction without the assistance of favoring positions. If you extend the arms sidewise and reach far out with both hands (or both elbows), then the shoulder-blades simply have to move away from each other. The test of your control is whether or not you can stand with the arms hanging limp at your sides, and then spread the shoulders apart, by merely willing them to move.

Again, while you will very soon learn to thus spread the blades apart (or. what is easier, to squeeze them together), you will have some trouble in learning to raise and lower them.

Undoubtedly, it helps you to get this power of up-and-down movement if you first move the shoulders in those sidewise circles. That is, move the points of the shoulders, since the shoulder-blades, being fastened to the shoulder-joint, have their position affected by every movement of that joint. And just as soon as you can move the shoulder-blades in that way—then you must learn to keep the shoulders themselves motionless, and make the shoulder-blades circle around apparently of their own will and volition.

Perhaps your shoulders will move a little at first, especially when you spread the blades; but if you stick at it you will advance in control until, when either sitting or standing, you can make the blades travel in circles; or lift them up, or depress them. It is a queer sensation, and gives you a feeling of new power. It affords a means of exercise for muscles which are rarely used: it will help straighten round shoulders, because when you move the blades in every possible way you are bound to use every muscle in the upper part of the back.

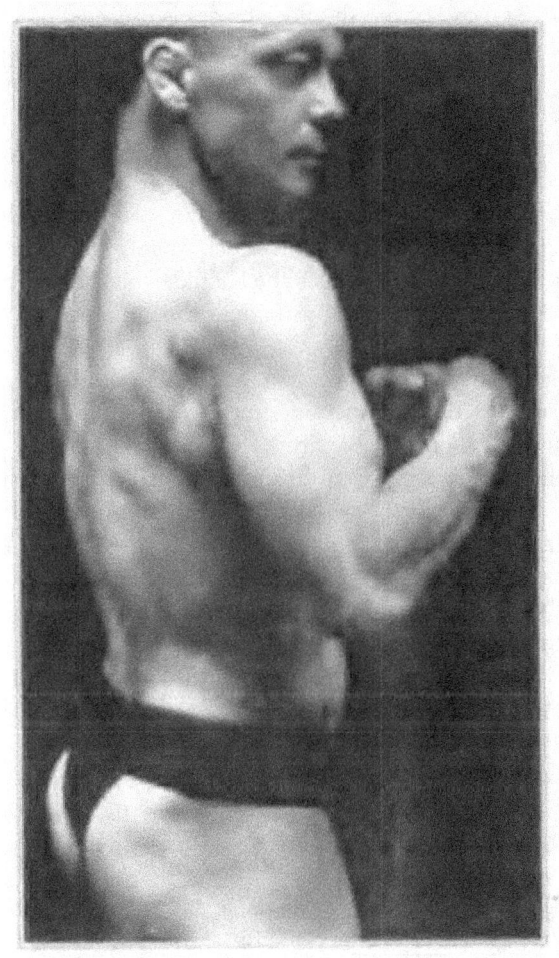

Рис. XII

The raising of the shoulder-blades is caused, as you know, by a contraction of the trapezius muscle. In Figures VIII and IX (August) this full contraction of the trapezius is shown. This stunt is just as spectacular when viewed from the side. It is done as follows: Turn the right side towards your mirror. Clasp the hands lightly in front of you, and then spread your shoulders far apart, as in Figure XII. which, of course, makes the shoulder-blades lie flat against the ribs, and thus flattens the upper back.

Then pass quickly to Figure XIII and again back to Figure XII (which is the same as doing Figures III and IV) but with the arms lowered. The flexing of the trapezius makes both shoulder-blades project as in Figure XIII (or as in Figure IX, both poses being the same). Repeat this several times in succession, as quickly as you can. The effect will be almost as though you had a small wing on your back, and that you were moving it as a bird does in flying. Almost all the exhibitionists include this stunt in their posing acts. Although you are not apt to do any public posing, you should include this in your practice because it helps to give you control; the power of voluntary movement of one of a pair of muscles.

You will find as you advance in this game that when there are a pair of muscles—one on either side of the medial line, (i.e., a right and a left) it is easiest to flex them simultaneously. And that it requires a new degree of concentration and control before you can relax one of the pair and make the other work independently.

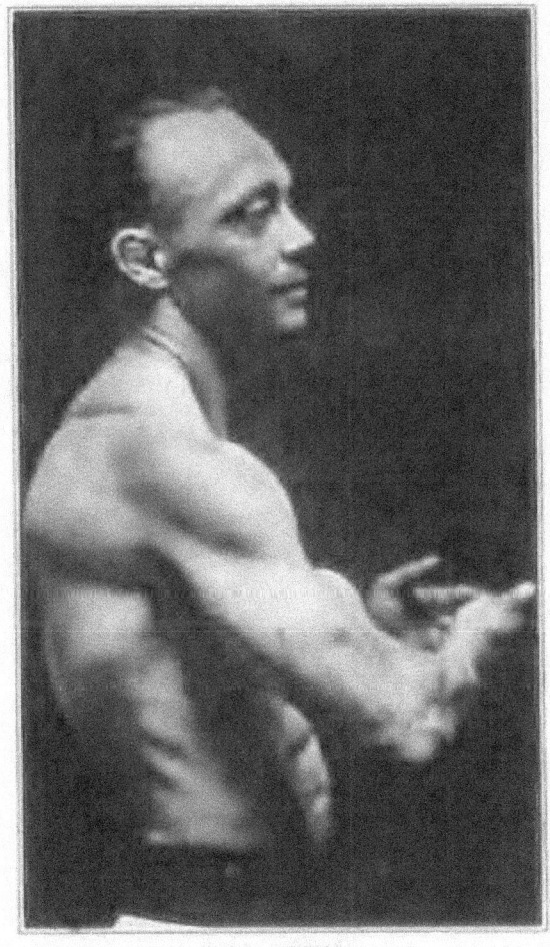

FIGURE XIII

Attached to the ribs are a set of muscles known as the serratus magnus, which are attached at their rear ends to the inside of the shoulder-blades— pass between the shoulder-blades and the ribs— and are fastened at their front ends to the ribs themselves. You can see them in Figure XIV on either side of the chest. In most men they are so little developed that they do not affect the surface form, but in powerfully developed men they are very prominent. You will see them outlined on the bodies of many of the ancient statues, particularly when the subject is represented in vigorous action.

(These muscles appear on the sides of the chest as a set of digitations—resembling a row of saw teeth.)

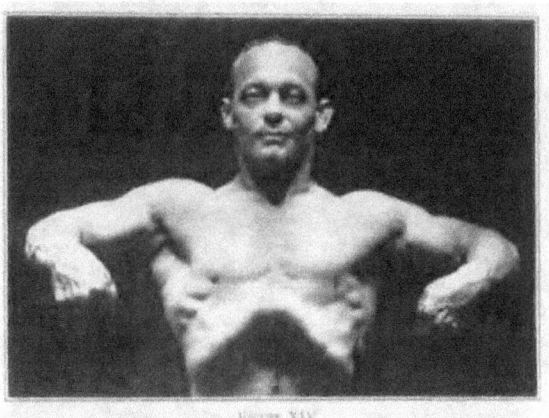

FIGURE XIV

These muscles are involved in the control of the shoulder-blade, since when the chest is inflated and the ribs fixed in position the contraction of the serratus magnus muscle spreads the blades. Hence it is almost impossible to control and display the serratus except when the chest is raised and the back spread as in Figure XIV. You have to think, not about the broad of the back muscles, but these serrate, tightening them as you force the shoulder-blades apart.

An easier way to get control is to raise the right arm over the head, raising the elbow high, as in Figure XV; lift and inflate the chest, and then spread the right side of the latissimus dorsi, i.e., move the right shoulder-blade away from the spine as you contract the serratus muscles.

The control of the serratus is mostly a "show stunt." Nevertheless it has its value in training the body. To obtain complete control of the body you have to learn to control every muscle and to relax every muscle. Besides which the serratus has a special value, in that it helps the mechanical, or muscular, expansion of the rib-box. It you hold the ribs fixed, the contraction of the serratus draws the shoulder-blades apart from each other. Therefore it follows that if you hold the blades firmly in their normal position, the serratus when it contracts (shortens) will necessarily lift the ribs and spread them further apart.

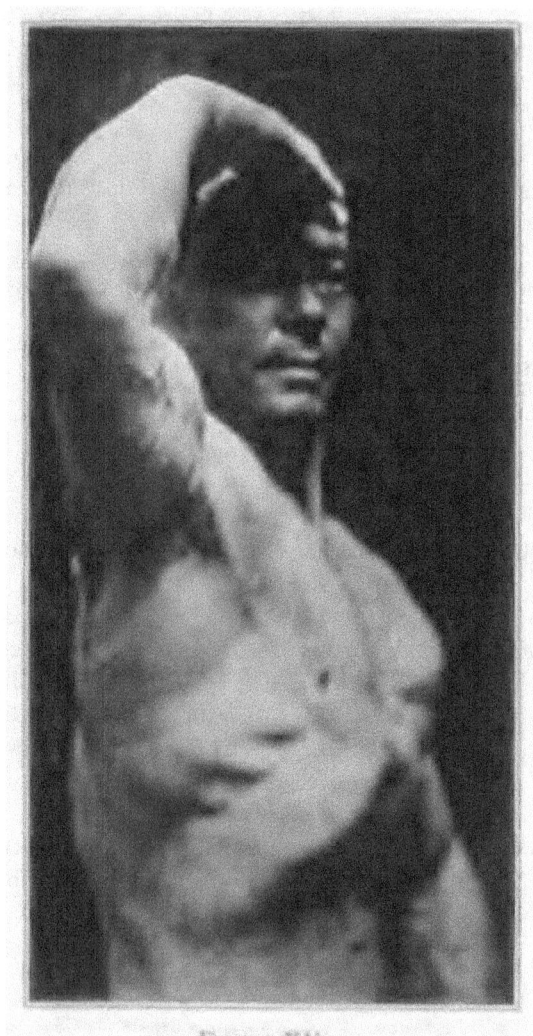

FIGURE XV

If you are a student of pictures of well-developed men, you may have noticed that these serratus magnus muscles are to be seen on the best developed men. You will see pictures of many beginners who show fine arms, good shoulder muscles and well- defined and clean-cut muscles on the breast, abdomen and upper back. But rarely do they reveal even an indication of the serratus muscle. Every athlete has them, of course, but in some cases these muscles are less developed than any others on the body—and in other cases the men may not know how to display them.

One reason these muscles are so neglected is that such a small part of them can be seen. Only their front parts he right under the skin: the greater part being overlaid by the shoulder-blades, and by other muscles. Again these muscles are but little affected by the ordinary arm-movements practiced by physical culturists. Their function is more to move the whole arm than to bend it at the elbow. One authority says that these are the muscles which furnish most of the power when a fencer makes a forward thrust. If that is so, they must be equally at work in a straight forward punch; and must help in throwing a ball.

Frequently you will find men with highly developed upper arms, and little or no serratus development. But if you find a man who has great latissimus muscles on the back, and great muscles at the sides of the waist, he is almost sure to have equally line serratus muscles.

One reason why this muscle-control practice is so valuable is because it brings you into close acquaintance with muscles which are neglected in other training systems. In the editorial in the first part of this issue you are given a few exercises for body muscles. The one shown in Figures VI and VII is an excellent developer of the serratus.

It is a well-known fact, to those who have specialized on the subject, that the experts—the professional or amateur "strong men"—can display the strength of two ordinary men. Not because their muscles are so much bigger than those of their weaker competitors, but because they use so many more of their muscles, and use the proper muscles at the right time. There are ways of doing feats by using the arms only—which mean small result, and great exertion—and there are other ways of reinforcing the arms with the strength of the body—muscles which control and actuate the upper arms; which transforms the stunt from a feat of arm strength, to a feat of bodily strength. In the latter case the exertion is far less and the results obtained are many times greater. The moral is that by learning how to use your body muscles you can double and perhaps triple the amount of force you can put in an arm movement.

There is nothing better than the muscle-control to bring your body muscles under your command.

CONTROL OF THE BREAST MUSCLES

One of the principal functions of the pectoral muscles— which are the superficial muscles of the breast—is to bring the arms forward and together. If you hold the arms straight and cross them in front of you, the pectoral muscles are contracted, and will rise in two hard mounds of muscle; that is, if the muscles have any development to start with.

The easiest way to learn to control them is to place the palms of the hands together as in Figure XVI and then press the hands together as hard as possible. That is bound to make the pectoral muscles contract to the limit. Try this in front of your mirror, and note that just as soon as you relax the pressure with the hands, the pectoral muscles relax and soften.

So, in order to get an alternate contraction and relaxation, all you have to do is to press, ease off, press again, etc. And every time you press you must concentrate your mind on the breast muscles; actually think into them.

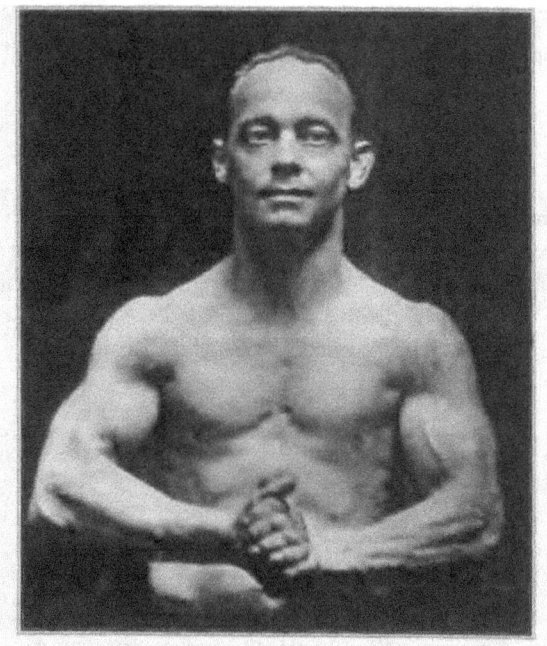

FIGURE XVI

The next step is (while still holding the arms in the position favorable to the contraction of the pectorals) to lessen the pressure with the hands, and to force the contraction by willpower. Do this by putting the thumbs together as in Figure XVII. Stand a minute with the breast muscles relaxed, as in that picture, and then press the thumbs together so as to harden and contract the pectorals as in Figure XVIII. You cannot press nearly as hard with the thumbs as with the palms; so, in order to get the same degree of contraction you must will the pectorals to flex.

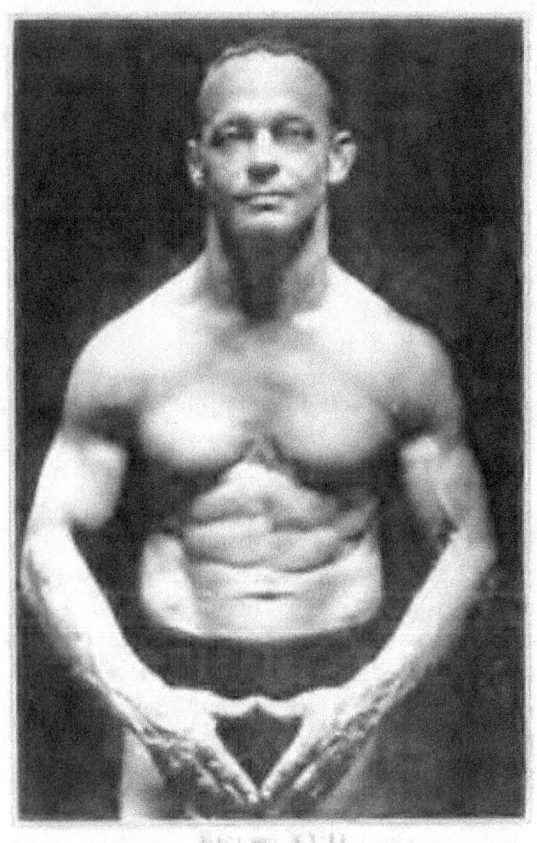

Figure XVII

After this try to make the pectorals flex by pressing the thumbs against the outside of the thighs. By pressing first on one side and then on the others, you can learn the alternate control of the pectorals.

The final step in control is to dispense entirely with the assistance of the arm position. Stand with arms hanging at the sides, and breast muscles relaxed as in Figure XIX. Then contract them by pure will-power and they should harden and flatten themselves as in Figure XX.

Every contraction should be followed by a movement of relaxation. You will make better progress if you contract and relax the breast muscles 15 or 20 times in rapid succession. Finally, when you have the muscles under complete menial control, you will be able in contract either pectoral muscle, while leaving its partner relaxed as in Figure XXI.

Of course you understand, that, like in all other control stunts, you must dispense with the mechanical assistance as quickly as possible Thus, as soon as you can get a good con traction of the pectorals by pressing the thumbs together, it is no longer necessary to press with the palms—and when you are able to flex them by will-power, you can dispense with the favoring arm position,—and be able to practice the stunt when sitting at ease reading a book. Just as it is said that Sandow used to take 15 minutes muscle-control exercise while reading his morning paper; using practically every one of his muscles one after the other, and yet without any perceptible movement of the whole body, or any alteration of his position. When you get to be an adept you will find that you can utilize muscle control in many different ways.

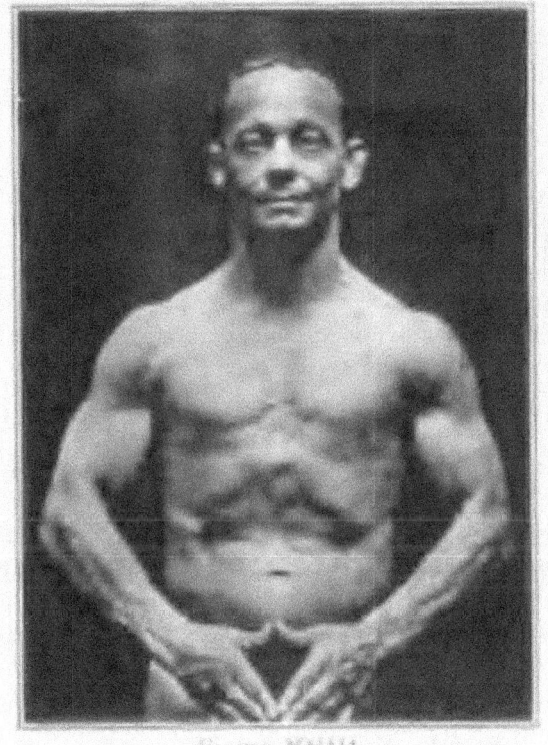

Figure XVIII

You can use it as a means of promoting blood-circulation and to get the muscles exercised and limbered up, as Sandow did. This feature has a great appeal to those who have to conserve their strength. It is possible to exercise every important group of muscles in a few minutes' time, and to further have the advantage of an entire freedom from fatigue.

You can employ it to increase your mastery of the body as a whole; which, as before said, will give you an immense advantage in competitive games, and athletic exercises.

What is perhaps more valuable still, you can use it as a method of relaxation; of ridding yourself of that nervous tension which interferes with perfect performance in either work or sport. It is a great thing to be able to make your body do what you want it to do.

But some of you are almost sure to want to display your ability in this line, and to impress your fellow-athletes with the amount of your development, and your mastery over your muscles. And (this in answer to queries) later on you will be given display stunts. Those are combination-feats wherein you simultaneously control several groups of muscles. Naturally, you first have to learn I0 contract the separate group. If you are wise, you will be patient and not attempt combination stuff too early in the game. Get each set of muscles under complete domination of your will before you try the complicated stuff.

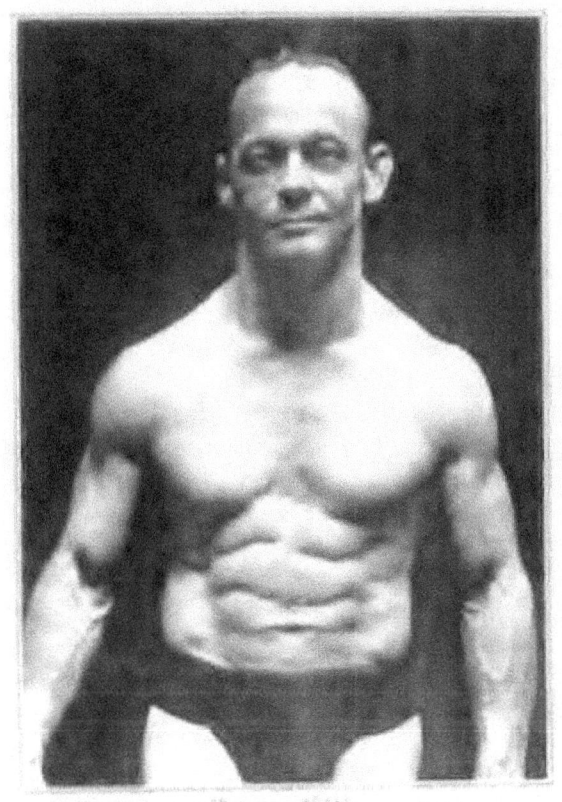

Figure XIX

Of course, I do not know (as yet), just how far you
expect to go with this control business. But I will
make a little prophecy right here, which is that
there is nothing like the combination stunts to
make you dissatisfied with your own shape and
development: that is, if you are honest with

yourself. After doing a simultaneous-control "pose" and mentally comparing your image in the mirror with the photo of Arco, Sandow or some other master doing a similar muscle pose, you will become resentful of your lack of shape and control. Well! If you persist you can get just as remarkable control as they have; and perhaps nearly, or quite, as much muscle. Although I will not say that you will ever get their beauty of form. Muscle-control is a help, an immense help, but it is not enough in itself to make the whole body grow to its natural limit of size, beauty and vigor.

I confess that these combination poses, fascinate me (Calvert) especially when I can persuade Arco into trying a new one, or surprise him in some position which reveals the muscles in a new way.

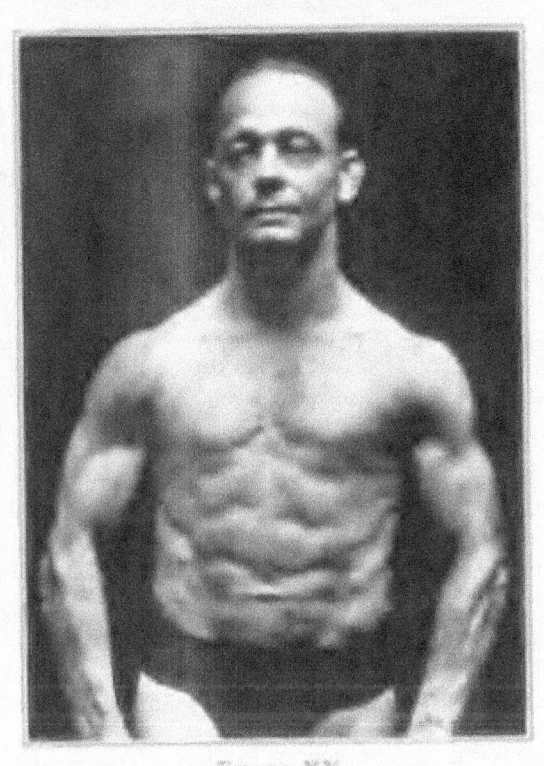

Figure XX

Sometimes I feel sorry for you fellows who have to read these articles. You have to listen, whether or no, to my particular enthusiasms. In the last few months I have been especially interested in the development and the possibilities of the back. So, when Arco is posing I am forever asking him to do back poses. Figure XXII is one of his latest. Here is a combination control stunt for you! He has the shoulders spread and the lower points of the shoulder-blades rotated outwards. To attain to that position he had to utterly relax his trapezius muscles, with the odd result that the upper fibres of both trapezius seem to merge into one band of muscle; resembling a scarf draped around his neck. Also the latissimus—(broad of the back) muscles are relaxed and hanging of their own weight.

In Figure XXIII, where Arco looks as though he was praying, that the posing session was over, the trapezius is relaxed from top to bottom and is so softened in outline that you can barely make out the characteristic kite-shape—the trapezius—which gives this pair of muscles their name. By drawing the shoulder joints forward he has made himself very broad across the back. The latissimus muscles are mildly flexed. The extraordinary thing is how he is able to apparently lift the latissimus off the underlying erector spinae muscles, at the back of the waist. The deep shadows there are partly due to the top-light and partly to the flexing muscles.

Figure XXIV was an idea of Mr. Scott's. He watched Arco doing a hand-stand, and became fascinated by the play of the back muscles, which assumed different outlines as they flexed in the effort to life the legs aloft. Finally, he decided that this particular pose gave the most unusual effect. Arco accommodatingly did the handstand several times in succession, until Scott caught him at the right instant. Certainly it is a new way of showing the back muscles at work. The latissimus shows plainly enough, but evidently the hardest work was being done by the erector muscles—these two cables alongside the spine, at and just above the waist line. Some necessity of balance makes these muscles merge into the external oblique muscles at the sides of the waist.

What would have interested you was the ability of Arco to stop at any point in the act of raising the hips and legs, and then holding his body immovably in balance. He, himself, said that that was practical muscle-control; which he considered an infinitely more valuable possession than the ability to show the muscles when posing.

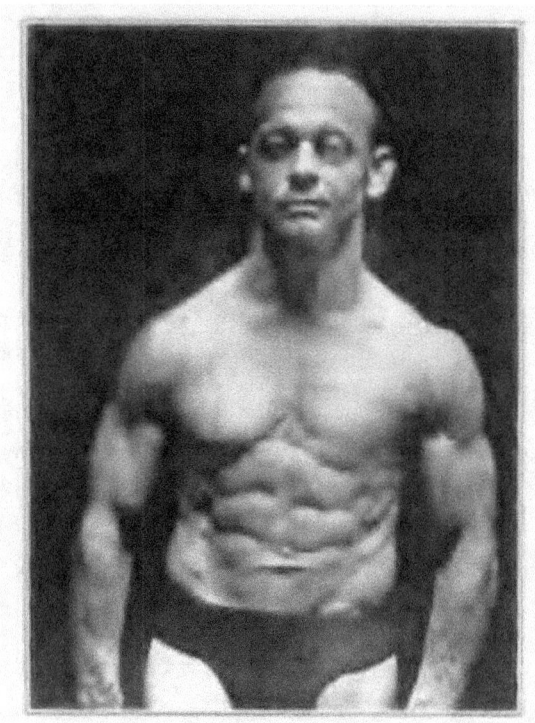

Figure XXI

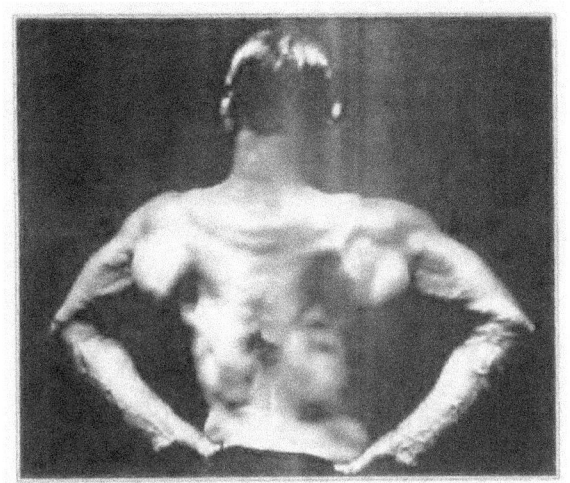

Figure XXII

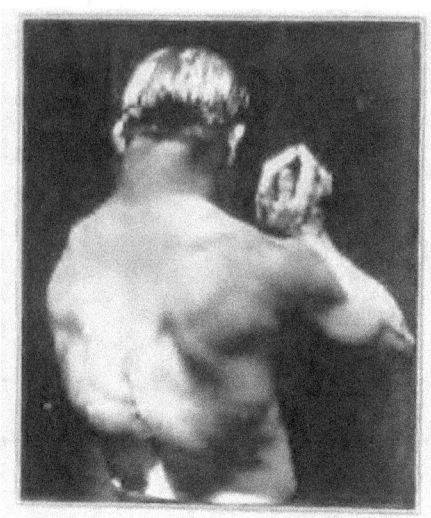

FIGURE XXIII

On submitting the foregoing to Arco, I got a general approval: together with one or two corrections (which have been made): and a reminder that I am not sufficiently emphasizing the necessity of complete relaxation, before and between contractions. He says that one can get a much higher degree of contraction if one starts with the muscle utterly relaxed; and that it is like putting the gear shift of your engine into neutral before starting the motion.

I can see his point, and how it applies to both practice and exhibition. When making several repetitions in practice you actually lose energy unless you do fully relax. Remember that the contraction is caused by a nerve impulse: that if, after contracting the muscle, you relax it only part way, then you are under a reduced but still continuous strain, and you have just that much less nerve-force to put into the next-contraction.

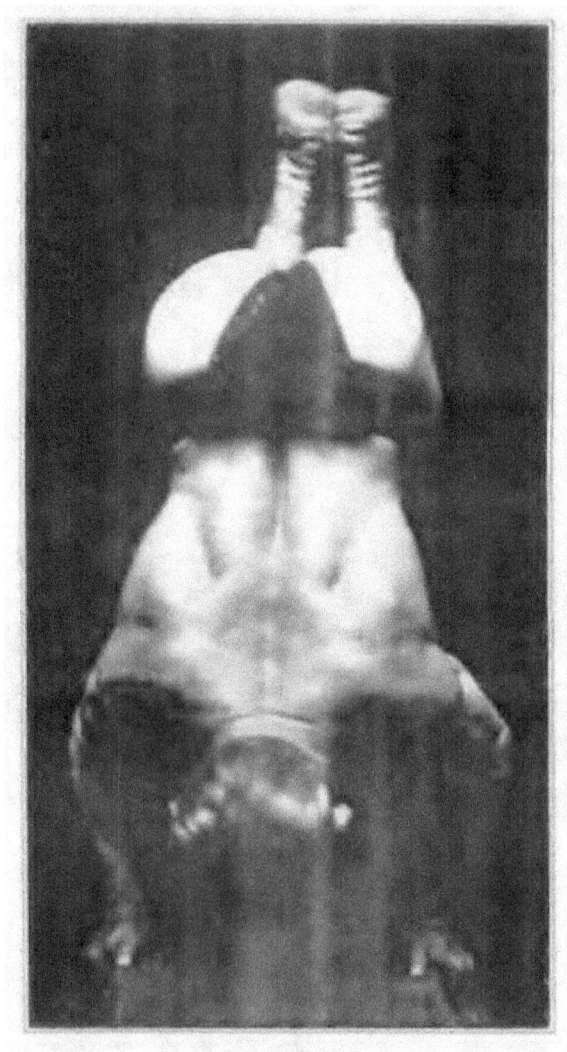

Figure X-XX

In exhibitions of muscle-control the complete relaxation becomes absolutely necessary. For the very object is to show your power t o increase the size of the muscles at will. If you start a stunt with a set of muscles utterly relaxed, and then contract them to the utmost, the change in the size, the shape, and the position of those muscles is something startling. Whereas if you start with the muscles already partly contracted, then the difference between partial and full contractions is obviously smaller. This makes itself very apparent when a control stunt is repeated rapidly and several times in succession. If the alternate contractions and relaxations are complete, the muscles alter greatly in appearance, and seem as though they were alive: if the relaxation is only partial, the effect is more like a mild twitching.

LESSON THREE

IN THE September lesson I told you that before attempting combination control feats it would be necessary for you first to learn to control the separate groups of muscle.

It was my intention to follow the back, and breast, control, with a lesson in the control and display of the arm-muscles. Instead, I am going to give you a sort of general lesson, including back, breast, arm and combination-movements.

The reason for the change of plan is that I was so lucky as to get hold of a motion-picture-film of my co-author, Mr. Arco. In swinging around the circuit Arco reached Los Angeles in early summer. In that city he is a great favorite, not only with the theatre-going public, lint also with many of the movie stars themselves. A particular pal of Arco's is Richard Talmadge; and, on the invitation of the latter. Arco visited Talmadge's studio and did his famous posing-act before the camera.

The result is that you, as readers of BODY MOLDING get the privilege of studying enlargements from that film: some fourteen of which accompany this article.

Perhaps some of you have already seen the pictures on the screen of your local theatre. I understand the film is being displayed the week before Arco gives his show in person. If so, you had a treat.

According to his own account, this film was a source of surprise and instruction to Arco himself, he told me that when he first saw it "run off" he was astonished at his own actions and poses. "Why," he said, "I found that I did some things which I never knew that I did. I could see where some of my poses could be improved by closer attention to detail. And honestly there was some actually startling effects as I shifted my position; for which I deserve no credit, because I never strove for, nor expected to get, those effects."

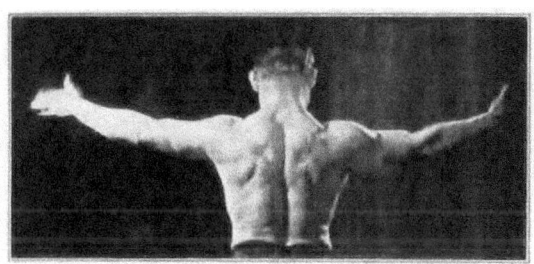

Figure XXV

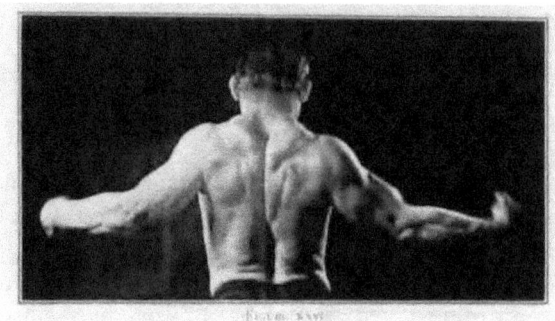

In the film there must be at least a couple of thousand separate pictures; each of them varying in the least trifle from the ones which precede and follow it. To go over the film inch by inch and pick out the precise poses you want is some job. If my pocketbook would stand it I would have the whole lot enlarged. As it was, I had to resist the temptation and try and select only the most unusual and instructive poses.

It is my experience that in "taking pictures" to show muscular display you rarely get as good a result when you have a mail stand up and "pose," as you do if you can get a snap-shot of him in action. I found that out long ago, when I used to take pictures of lifters, if I used a movie-camera and took a picture of a lift, then the pictures of the athlete actually exerting himself showed far more muscle than if I had the man pose for a "still" in a regular studio. In a "set pose", no matter if the athlete was handling a genuine Weight, he never looked as well, nor showed as much muscle as he would show in the actual lifting.

In muscle-poses the difference is not as great: but still these enlargements, being of pictures reeled off as Arco was passing without a pause from one pose to the next, show us many things we would never see in "stills." Furthermore the film contained a lot of positions, which I, for one, would never have thought of attempting to take if I had an athlete before the ordinary camera. Some of the very finest poses in Arco's film are the ones which he has never attempted before a "still" camera. Among them are ones which give you a better idea of the man, his proportions, and development, than others in which he is frankly striving for spectacular effects.

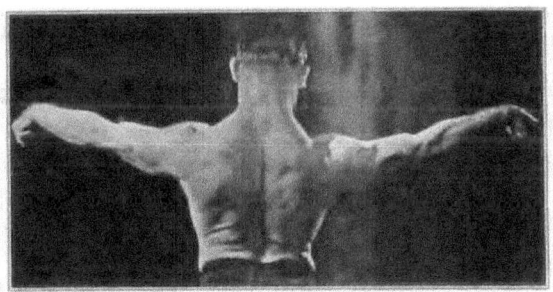

FIGURE XXVII

To start with there is Figure XXV, which will make Arco exclaim in vexation. It is one of those relaxed transition poses. It is half-way between Figures I and II in the August issue. His back is relaxed and normal. There is just as much contraction in the shoulder muscles as is caused by holding the arms horizontal. The blades are pressed slightly together. The lower half of his back is partly contracted, and his arms utterly relaxed. This shows the man exactly as he is when is not trying for display; just as he looks when Mr. Scott says "Arco! Hold out your arms so I can see whether all of you is on this plate."

As an "effect," it looks more impressive to me than when he is doing feats of extreme control; it is so symmetrical and gives such an impression of power. What Arco will object to is the arms. You see, he forgot himself for a moment. He has his right arm palm-up, which brings the biceps into profile and makes the relaxed triceps hang of its own weight, thus showing the relaxed arm to the best advantage. His left arm is almost palm-down, which rotates the arm so that it appears narrow. There is actually not much difference in the size of the left and right arms. Had the left palm been up the left arm would have been just as impressive as its mate.

Figure XXVI shows the shoulder-blades slightly raised and then jammed tightly together; making the back narrow, but displaying muscles which are not prominent when tile blades are spread apart. Note how in this pose, Arco has done just what he did with his arms in Figure XXV: given his right arm all the best of it by rotating it into the most favorable position for display.

In Figure XXVII both arms look just the same size, because they are held in the same position. Here is a back-pose which you seldom see. The shoulders are spread as far apart as possible, and also are strongly depressed. As a consequence the back looks very short, has a sharp taper to the waist, and while there is not much display of muscle across the shoulders, there is evidence of tremendous muscles across the broad of the back from the armpits down to the waist line. Figure XXVII is an excellent illustration for one part of the "shoulder circling" taught in August.

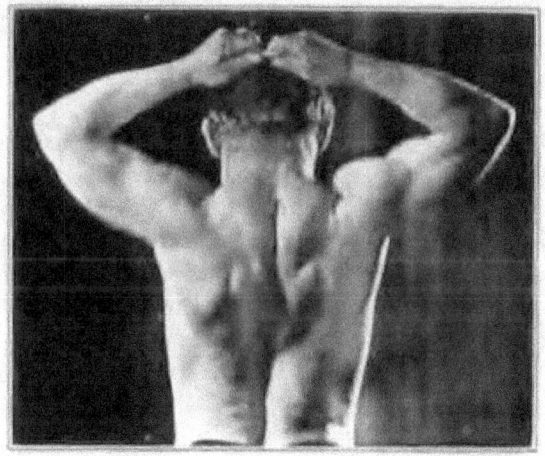

FIGURE XXVII

Remember that you were told to stand with arms outstretched, and then to move the points of the shoulders in circles. Some readers misunderstood the directions. They described fore-and-aft circles with the shoulders: that is they moved the shoulders up, front, down, back up—for the forward circle: or just the reverse for the backward circle.

That helps as a shoulder loosener, but it is not the movement described. You should move the shoulders up, apart, down, together, up. etc., or down, apart, up, together, etc. You move the shoulders in sidewise circles; not front-and-back circles. Figure XXVII shows the shoulders apart and down. Figure XXVIII shows them up and together. Neither of these poses was intended to illustrate the circling movement, but they will give you an understanding of the terms we have to use in describing upper-back movements.

Figures XXVIII and XXIX are m close sequence in the film, XXVIII is just before Arco starts to do the sidewise projection of the shoulder blades. In XXIX the shoulder-blades are moving away from each other, and he is putting some tension in the arms and shoulders. From XXIX he will continue until he gets the full projection: as in Figure VI.

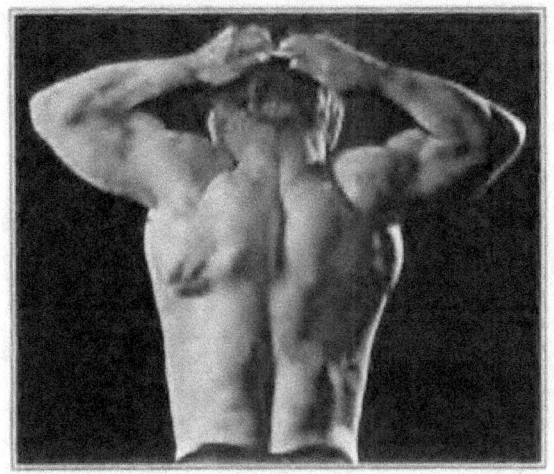

FIGURE XXIX

The difference between Figure XXVIII and Figure VI is startling. Arco goes from one position to the other so rapidly that the eye does not register the intermediary stage (XXIX), but the camera has caught it for us.

It will assist in your control if you will practice going quickly from XXVIII to VI: repeating several times. Do not forget that the shoulders must he raised before the shoulder-blades can he projected In XXVIII there is quite a space between the shoulders and the ears. In XXIX and VI the shoulders have been elevated so much that the deltoids touch the ears. In VI Arco has his upper-arms and deltoids flexed. It is not necessary for you to do that while practicing. An exhibitionist has to do it even when directing the eyes of the audience to one particular muscle, he can not afford to let the other muscles go lax.

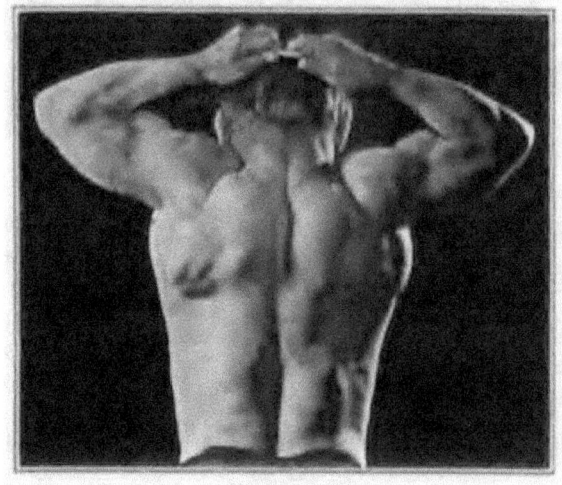

FIGURE XXIX

Figure XXX is the front view of pose VII. Arco has increased the effect by retracting the abdomen and elevating the diaphragm: just as you were taught to do in one of the special exercises in the "costal breathing" articles.

If you have been practicing since you read the August issue, you should have already gotten control of the shoulder-blades, and of the diaphragm. So if you wish to, you can combine the two; as Arco is doing in Figure XXX. It will be a good test of your ability in simultaneous control.

Figure XXXI is shown for no reason at all, except that I happen to like it. It has little to do with this muscle-control work. In examining the film I chanced to notice this, in a row of pictures where he was turning his back to the audience. It is nothing remarkable as a muscle display, but it does show Arco's shape; his square shoulders, his deep chest; his natural muscularity. The arms, shoulders, and lack are slightly tensed; his hands are bent back so as to show the muscles on the outside of the fore arms. There is a grand body for you: enough of everything and not too much of anything. The chest looks square—almost box-like—but it is the rounded squareness that marks the torso of the athlete.

Figures XXXII, XXXIII and XXXIV are poses which you should try and imitate; not because they are striking as poses, but so that you can get practice in displaying several different muscles at the same time.

In Figure XXXII almost every muscle above the waist is flexed. You can start by contracting the trapezius and pectoral muscles. Those two great humps of muscle from the shoulder-points to neck are caused by the contraction of the trapezius. You were taught that control in August (Figure VIII). The breast-muscles are contracted in XXXII. You were taught control of the pectorals in the September lesson. If you can successfully display both trapezius and pectoral muscles, then lean a little bit forward (as Arco is doing), and flex the abdominal muscles into ridges. Never mind about the deltoids, arm and side-muscles; be satisfied with controlling three groups if you can.

Figure XXXIII is similar to Figure VIII but is harder to do; for in XXXIII Arco has flexed the trapezius, deltoids, pectorals, abdominal, and the arm-muscles; too much for a beginner like yourself to try.

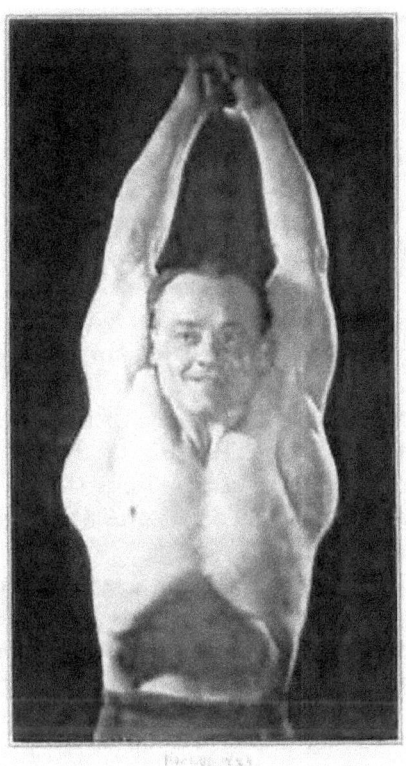

Figure XXXIV is one of the positions which make it easy to control the pectorals (breast muscle). Instead of pressing the hands, or thumbs together at the level of the waist line. Arco has raised his arms, brought his shoulders forward, and is pressing his knuckles together. This arm position (shoulders forward, remember) has the effect of lifting the breast-muscle away from the ribs. If you control them (alternately flex and relax them) their movement is of considerable range and rather spectacular. You can add this to the exercises given in the September lesson. It will help you to control the breast muscles in another way.

One thing in Figure XXXIV you must not miss: the front edge of the left latissimus dorsi (broad of the back) muscle, which looks, as though it were wrapped around the left edge of the body. That is a result of moving the shoulders forward. Both the breast and back muscles are fastened to the bones which make the shoulder joint. Therefore when the shoulders are pushed forward, the breast muscles are relaxed, and the back muscles stretched. It is very seldom that you see both effects in one picture.

Figure XXXV is Arco's own individual version of the "arms up" pose. Nobody else can quite equal him in this position. In the first place his control of the upper-arm muscles is so great that it is not necessary for him to bend hi- arms all the way in order to make his biceps prominent, he I tend- the arms only half-way at the elbows; sacrifices only a little of the biceps, but gains by being able to make the triceps bigger. He bend- his hands inward so as to show the wrist flexors, he raises his shoulders, which make the deltoids stands out beautifully, he spreads the shoulders apart so a- to impart a taper to the body. The spread of the shoulders enables him to display the serratus magnus. And lastly he is doing that odd stunt known as the "one sided"

74

control of the abdomen. The diaphragm has been lifted; but it should be noted that the right half of the abdominal muscle is relaxed, while the left half is contracted into a rope (compare this to the picture in August, page 47 where both halves of the abdominal muscle are contracted). Count up and you will see that Arco is simultaneously controlling at least eight different muscle-groups; has to think of eight things at once.

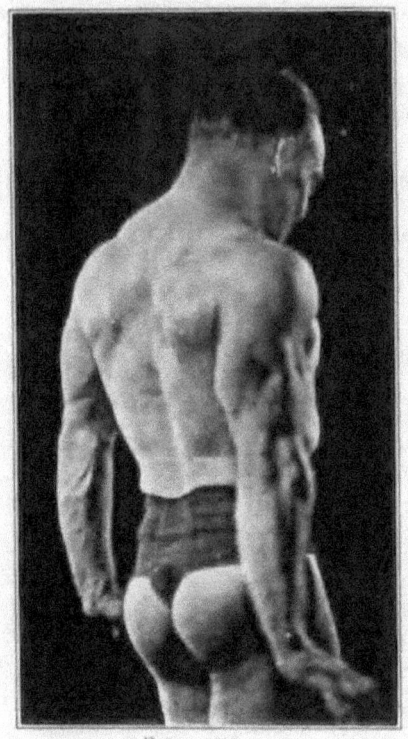

Figure XXXI

Difficult as that may sound; it is no harder for him than it is for you to harden the biceps alone. As you gain in knowledge and control, you will get Arco's ability to control all of your muscles singly, in groups, or any other way you may wish to use them.

Not only in posing mind you. That is only part—the smaller part. The great thing is to learn to make your body do what you want it to do, and when you want it to.

Figures XXXVI, XXXVII and XXXVIII are found fairly close together in the film (there are a few between XXXVI and XXXVII, and maybe two dozen more between that and XXXVIII. You know it takes a foot or so of film to record a slow movement.) Anyway Arco first holds his arm out to the side as in XXXVI—putting very little tension on the muscles. Then he very slowly bends the arm; slowly, because he knows that it fascinates the audience to see that ever-growing biceps. XXXVII shows the arm one-quarter bent; he is putting the tension into the biceps. In XXXVIII he has completed the movement, and his biceps is at its very biggest.

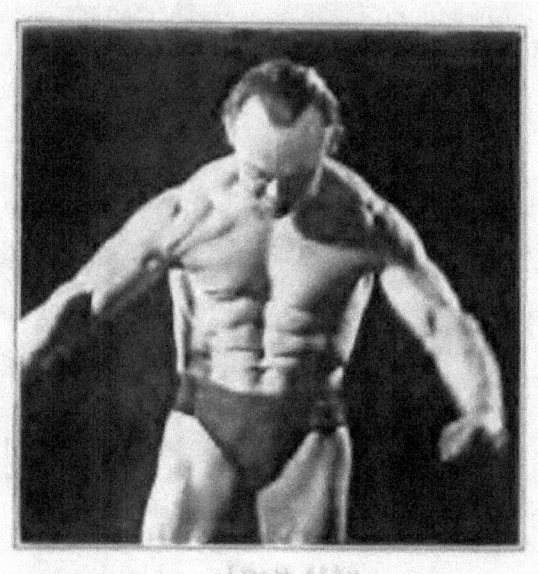

The last three pictures furnish an object lesson of the methods of an expert. Note that in the one where his arm is extended and relaxed, that his body is similarly relaxed; hardly a muscle shows on it. In the second where the arm is partly bent, with its muscles tensed, there is the same degree of tension in the body muscles; they all commence to stand out. And in that last one, where the arm is fully flexed, the shoulder and body muscles reflect the same tension. The body now shows a lot of light and shade—the outline of the muscles.

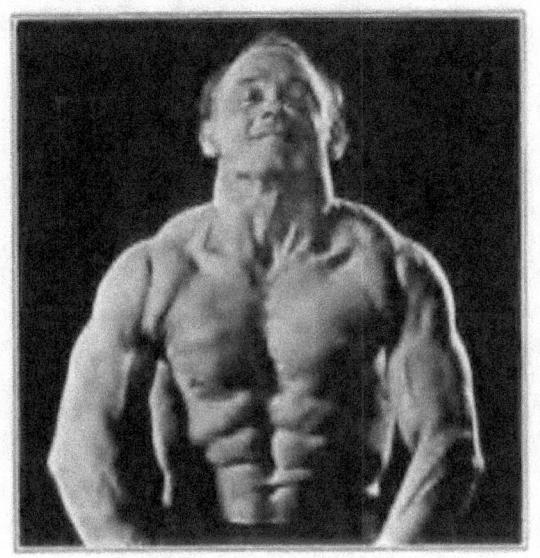

FIGURE XXXIII

No one seeing Arco in his usual attire would take him for anything other than what he actually is—a remarkably proportioned and extremely powerful-looking man. It is utterly impossible to overlook his chest and shoulders. More than that his strength is evinced by the way he carries himself, the way he moves, and his every little action. I have never seen him slouch whether standing or walking; never seen him slump when sitting. In fact I think it would be an effort for him to sit with an arched spine the way many people do. His muscles seem to hold him properly erect at all times.

Consequently he cannot help having the shape which goes with such erectness.

I called your attention to the size of his chest. I know that in his time he has taken a bit of exercise of various kinds. But then, I know a number of middle-aged amateurs who have exercised just as long and just as hard perhaps a hundred times more—than the average amateur knows. The exercise he has taken has permanently improved his build; given him such a shape that he no longer has to exercise to keep that shape. In all the time I have known him I have never once seen him with his chest caved in. No wonder his chest is big. The way he holds himself insures that.

I am interested in this muscle-control scheme, just as Checkley was interested in it. But the feature that appeals to me is that muscle-control will gradually lead you to bodily-control. At present there are some readers of this magazine who are unable to master the niceties of posture, because if such individuals learn all the different stunts in this series of lessons, it will help them to bring the entire body under the subject of the will; and thus render easy the mastery of posture.

Then there are other beneficial results, which come from the practice of muscle-control; things like the loosening up of stiffened joints; the increase of development coming from extreme contractions: and the reduction of surplus flesh. It may sound odd to speak of muscle-control as a waist-reducer, but when you come to practice some of Arco's stunts for the control of the abdominal and side muscles, you will find (if you are big-waisted) that in mastering these stunts you literally burn up the fat which impedes the muscular contraction and display.

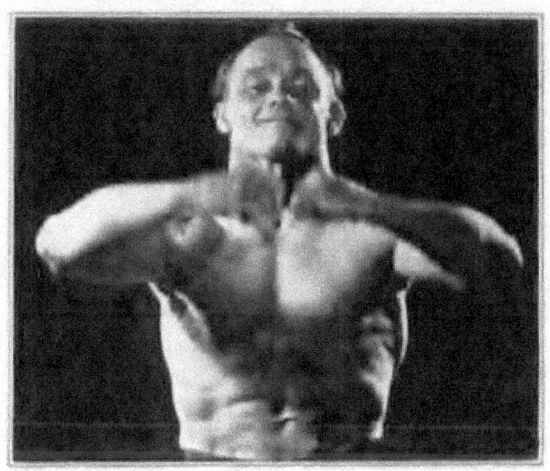

I have often thought that the immense popularity of muscle-control in Europe—muscle-control as a means of exercise—was that its practice created shape, reduced flesh and brought development, without any attendant fatigue; and, what is just as important, without it being necessary to go to any special place to practice, or to set aside any special time for practice.

No two people think exactly alike.—Arco and myself for example. He uses the display feature of muscle-control as a part of his stage work; nevertheless he considers its really important function to be the control it gives over the body in two other ways; the instant control which enables a man to both utilize his strength in athletics, gymnastics, or anything which requires skill or strength.—speed or dexterity, and the greater self control which strengthens character. While I value control one of his direct means of acquiring the shapely, supple figure which in itself is a guarantee of vigorous and continued health.

It took me hours and hours to go over the movie-film. I got a lot of pleasure out of it, but, as I have already said, I appreciated more the unstudied poses (where he was moving from one display to another) than I did the formal display—poses with which I have so long been familiar.

In exactly the same way when the two of us go to Mr. Scott's studio, in order that Arco shall make some "still" poses, it is work for all three of us. But Arco who docs the posing,—patiently assumes one position after another for perhaps three successive hours, comes away fresh as a daisy and just as gay as he always is; while Scott and I are tired out.

My pleasure on those occasions comes from watching Arco between poses. The instant the camera-shutter has clicked he relaxes and walks around the studio, continuing our conversation. Then you see the man at his best. He never saunters—he is too much alive to ever saunter. He paces up and down the room, easily, just as a leopard paces his cage. That is the kind of a moving picture I like. He presents a series of unstudied poses: each one of them perfect by reason of his symmetry, his poise and the easy flow of his satin-smooth muscles.

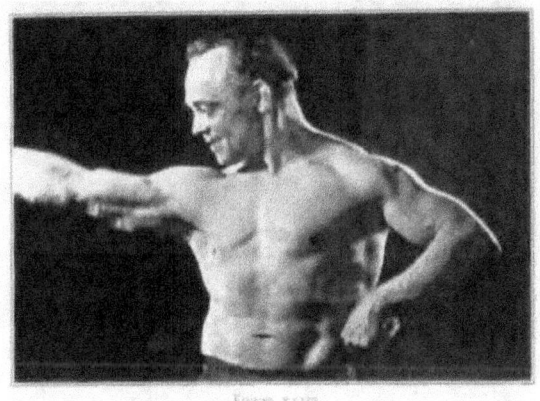

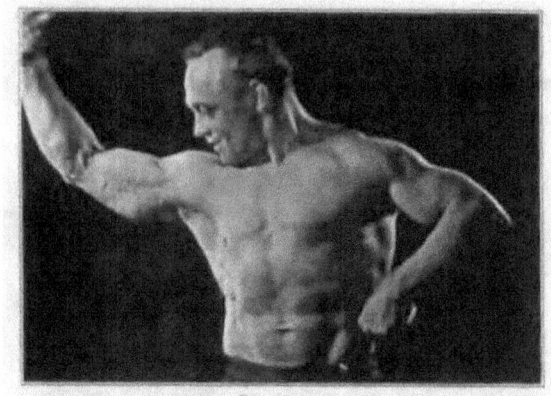

FIGURE XXXVII

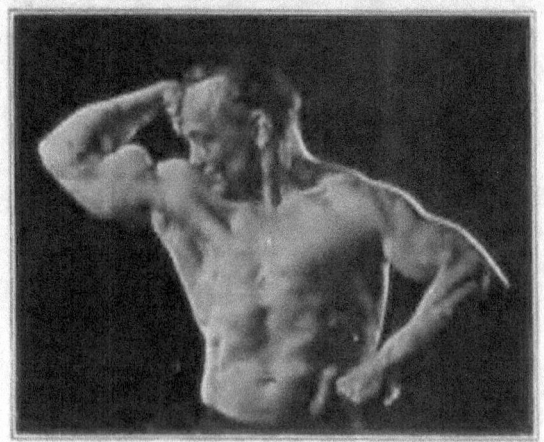

FIGURE XXXVIII

The only way I have of learning how you are impressed by the articles in BODY MOLDING is by the letters you write me. I constantly receive letters discussing the question of breathing; frequently get communications about the details of walking; and. of course, many requests for instruction about posture in all its aspects. But so far I have hail surprisingly few reports from those who are trying these muscle-control stunts. I assume that a great many of you must have at least tried them, even if you are not practicing; them regularly. If such is the case why not give the rest of us the benefit of your experiments; let us learn of your successes, and perhaps profit by your failures.

Because if you have been unsuccessful — have not been able to make your various muscles contract at will, or have not been able to make the different parts of your body protrude as they should in response to such muscular contraction—it means that the fault is more likely to be ours than yours. It may be that our directions have not been clear enough. On the other hand it is equally possible that you have not given enough study to the instructions; have overlooked one little detail which is necessary to the successful accomplishment of the stunt.

For instance, let us go back to the most spectacular of the stunts already described—the sidewise projection of the shoulder blades shown in Figure VI. This position is so unusual and causes so much surprise and amazement to the beholders, that most beginners try to learn it first of all. Now in the direction in the August lesson it said "raise the arms straight above the head (reaching as high as possible)" but not until later did we explain that it was necessary to force the arms upward in order to pull the lower points of the shoulder blades from under the top edges of the latissimus muscles. Possibly some who read the former, bypassed the latter, and therefore did not realize the absolute necessity of forcing the arms and shoulders up, before trying to spread the lower points of the blades to the sides. In many stunts there are details which are just as important, which you might overlook because they were not emphasized.

So if you get stuck write in and tell us so. We cannot guarantee individual letters in reply; be we can give further explanations in these articles. And if you have succeeded, tell us about the degree to which you have mastered the art; and send pictures in proof. We can use such reports and pictures for the encouragement of those who have not yet achieved control.

LESSON FOUR

LET us start with the most significant part of these series of stunts of arm control,—the litter relaxation between periods of contraction. Before, between, and after stunts Arco would indulge in an orgy of muscle-shaking. Letting his arms hang loosely at his sides he would start in to shake them slowly; then faster, and faster until his arms were a blur. The tremendous biceps and triceps muscles between his elbows and shoulders would literally flop about. He allowed them to go absolutely limp and flaccid; and as he vibrated the arms, the muscles seemed to be as loose as jelly. After that he would wring his hands, waving them about to relax the fore-arm muscles; doing it so rapidly that he seemed to have as many fingers as there are petals in a chrysanthemum. It was a curious exhibition; and would have surprised some of you who think that control of the muscles means only the ability to contract them to the limit: that and nothing more.

Once again I will say that Arco considers the ability to relax to be a higher art, and a more useful accomplishment than to be able to contract. He says that almost anyone can contract the arm muscles, harden them; but that too many physical culturists overemphasize the value of hard muscles; err on the side of always striving to make the muscle hard instead of trying to keep I them flexible. All muscles, he says, should be firm, but never actually hard unless in the act of contraction: as when actually at work nr purposely flexed for an instant's display. His own muscles, while remarkable for their size and contour, are just about as softly firm as those of a school-boy: have none of the rigidity which causes fatigue.

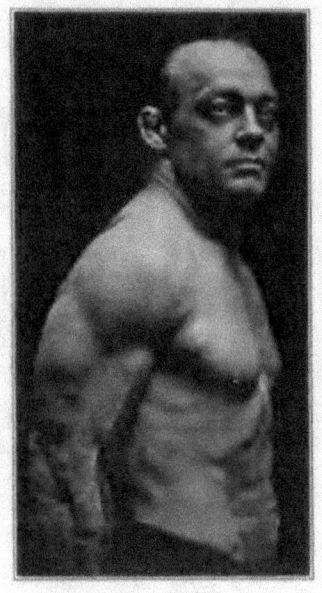

Plate XXXIX

From the muscle-control standpoint, relaxation affords both an opportunity for presenting contrast, and increases the ability of the muscle to contract by giving it a complete though momentary rest. Relaxation restores a jaded muscle. All the foregoing is said intentionally. Arco is very evidently convinced that I. who am doing the actual writing, do not say enough about cultivating the power to relax. He lectures me about it. "This muscle-control to the limit," he will say, "is hard work. Here I am making my arm muscles stand out. To do that I have to flex them hard, just as hard as though they had to overcome the resistance of a heavy weight. If I only flexed, flexed, flexed, my muscles would get still and slow just as they would if I made too many repetitions with a heavy weight. So I rest them and limber them." And again he would shake his arms.

In that connection it is interesting to study Figures XXXIX and XL illustrating the control of the triceps. That muscle, as it flexes, straightens the arm: brings the forearm in line with the upper-arm. Besides that it has another function; to draw the arm lip and back of the body.

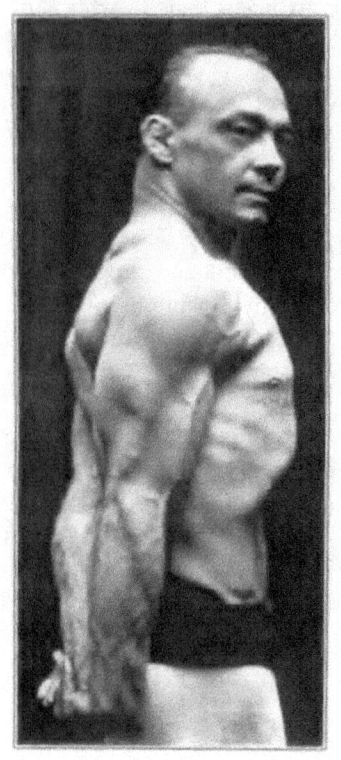

TAFEL XL.

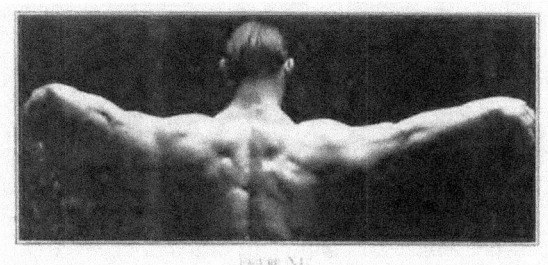

FIGURE XL

Therefore to place the muscles in the most favorable position for contraction (and the greatest ease of control) you must straighten the arms and move them back past the body until you can clasp the hand behind you. (Arco merely grasps the middle finger of the right hand with the thumb and forefinger of the left.) For the preliminary relaxation you allow the arms to bend a little at the elbows (as in Figure XXXIX) and then you straighten them, so as to hunch up the triceps into that sort of horseshoe-shape.

In the relaxed pose the triceps seems to present one unbroken flow of muscle all the way from the deltoid (shoulder) muscle down to the point of the elbow. In its flexed slate the length of the triceps seems to be reduced by at least one-third. It looks as though it started half way to the shoulder on the outside of the arm, and two inches above the elbow on the inside. It does shorten. To contract is to shorten. The flat space right above the elbow in Figure XL is the broad tendon of the triceps.

To contract the triceps vigorously you have to think into it. Straightening the aim is only part of the trick. You will make much better progress if you practice before a mirror so that you can watch the muscle. As you impress yon can omit the slight bend at the elbow. Hold the arm rigidly straight and alternately relax and contract by pure will-power. That will give you the effect of muscle rippling up and down the back of the arm, if you have an audience this stunt will astonish them: for while they are accustomed to see muscles flex as the limbs move, they wonder at a man's power to move his muscles while the limb itself is immovable.

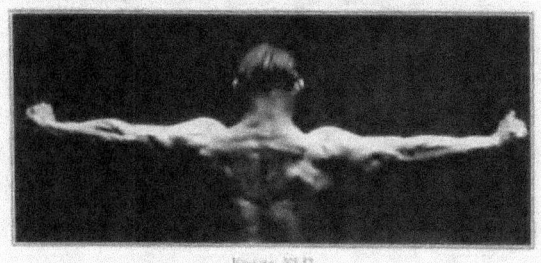

Figure XLII

But so far as appearance goes, which of the two pictures do you prefer? Is the flexed triceps in XI any more attractive than the relaxed arm in XXXIX? Or, although they are flexed, are the muscles in XI any more clean cut than those in XXXIX? To my mind the relaxed pose shows a far more impressive arm: the muscles are just as clean cut and even more shapely. There is the great test for you. How do you look when your muscles are relaxed? Have you enough shape and bulk to look well when you are not trying to make an impression? (Incidently, it might be mentioned that if a man's upper-arm is thin, it usually is because he lacks triceps development. If you use this stunt as an exercise and flex the triceps vigorously, you can add somewhat to the size of the muscle, and vastly improve the shape).

Practice at triceps-control should not be confined to one arm-position. You should be able to flex and display them any time the arm is held straight.

Figure XLI shows Arco with his arms relaxed; all the muscles soft, and the triceps hanging of its own weight. In XLII he has hardened actually all his arm muscles; gripped his hands making the forearm muscles stand out in cords; raised the shoulders so as to make the deltoids more prominent; and, particularly flexed the triceps (the biceps is hardly affected because in both pictures it is the position of relaxation).

(The hardening of all the muscles is not necessary. It happens that this "arms-out" is one of Arco's regular displays in his posing act, and when asked to flex the triceps he seems to automatically snap into his accustomed pose.)

In most cases where you wish to control the upper-arm muscles, it is a help if you first put some tension on the forearm muscle. To show the isolated control of the triceps, I asked Arco to make the pose XLIII, where the forearms and shoulders are limp and only the triceps contracted. It is much harder to do, but teaches a superior sort of independent control: also, it makes a good display stunt when you get so far that you can hold the arm out to the side, and then by successive contraction make the triceps literally hop about. The trick is to harden the triceps by contraction and then to relax quickly so that it falls into the hanging position. Should be repeated rapidly, and is much more showy when viewed from the front. (Another use for your mirror.)

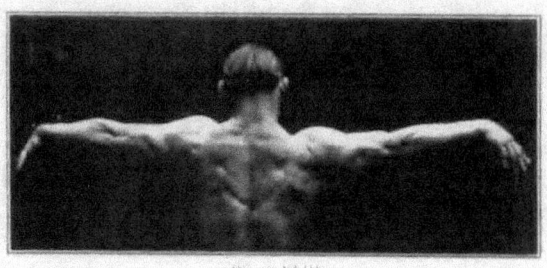

POSE XLIII

I introduced pose XLIV, not because it is one of the stunts.

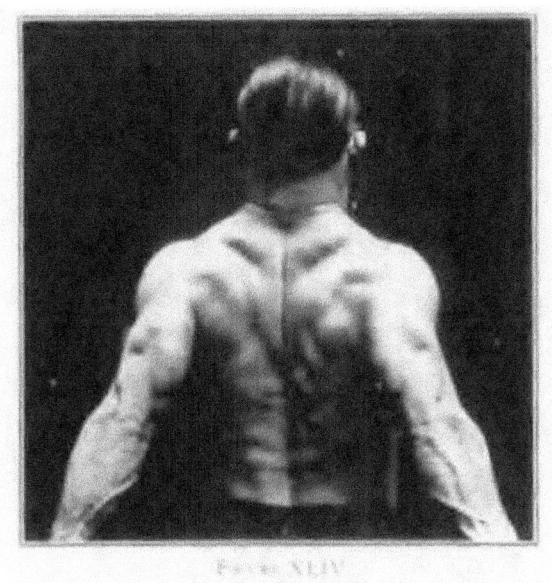

Plate XLIV

BICEPS

It seems as though it were superfluous to tell a physical-culturist how to display and control his biceps. If an exercise enthusiast can control no other muscle in his whole body, he can at least make his biceps obey his will.

Still it is surprising how many there are who fail to realize the full possibilities of control and display. If you wish to show the size of your whole arm, then it is all right to hold it by your side, with the elbow at the waist; but if it is the biceps you want to display, then the higher the elbow goes the more force you can put into the contraction and the more the muscle will rise up.

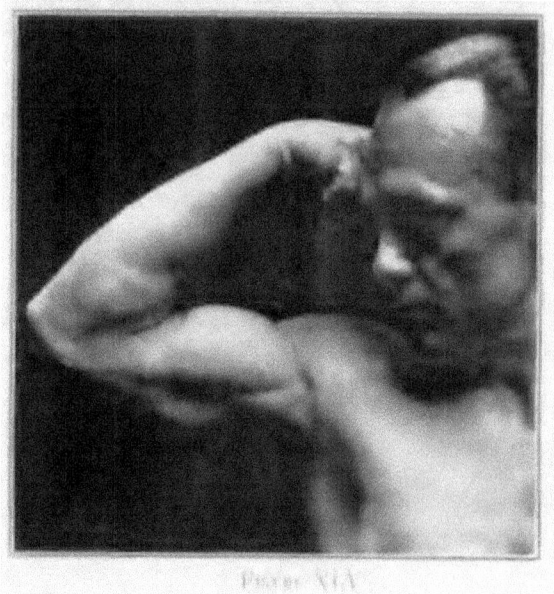

Plate XIA

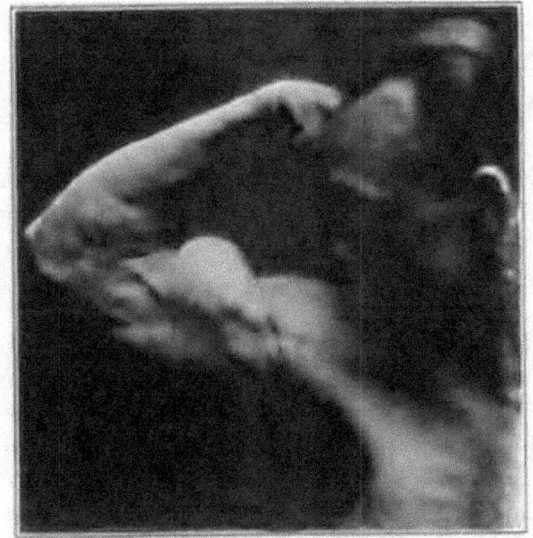

Figure XLVI

Now to go back a few paragraphs; to the men who do not know how to show their biceps. If that muscle is to be bunched up, balled-up, or whatever term you wish to use, the arm must be fully bent and the palm of the hand must be toward the shoulder.

If, with his arm in position XLVI, Arco should keep his upper-arm and forearm immovable and rotate his hand from knuckles-up to palm-up, then immediately the biceps would change its shape. The lump would become longer and not so high. Try it yourself. Get in position XLVI, palm down, make the bicep hump as much as possible and then rotate your hand to palm-up. Watch the lump go. Keep changing your hand from one position to another and the bicep will repeatedly change its shape. But no matter how you try you cannot keep it at its highest unless the palm is down. (Some physical culturists actually do not know that. When they show their biceps, they keep the palm pointing out, or up. Consequently the biceps never really bunches and they become convinced that their muscles are "long."

The reason is that the biceps at its lower end tapers to a tendon which is attached to the outer bone of the forearm. In the palm-down position that bone is close to the shoulder. When you reverse the hand to palm-up, you rotate the forearm on its own axis, alter the respective position of the forearm bones and increase the distance between the origin and insertion of the biceps.

The biceps has two heads. Two bellies that almost merge into one. The heads are attached by separate tendons to the shoulder blade.

Now listen. If you want to teach the biceps the position of ultimate contraction; practice flexing it with the elbow raised above the bead as in XLIX or even higher than that. Start with the arm as in XLVI, put all the tension on the biceps you can, raise your elbow and slide your fist down to the back of your neck. As the elbow rises the tension on the biceps will result in a painful cramp, and the bicep will hump up as it never has before. The reason, I believe, is that the forearm bone is actually nearer the shoulder blade, thus allowing the bicep to contract exceedingly. I may be wrong, perhaps some anatomist can give us a better explanation.

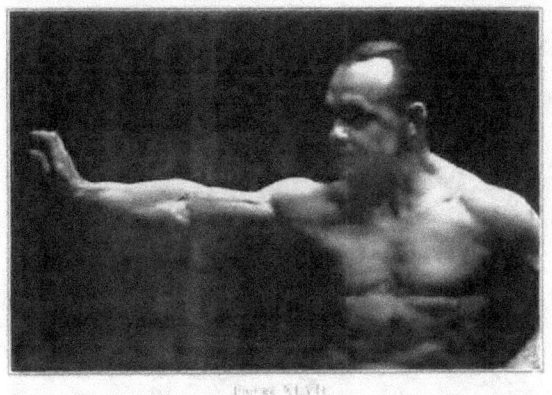

Plate XLVII.

The value of doing that "elbow up" is to educate the biceps' contractile power; it will assist you to bunch it up more in position XLVI and will increase your control of it.

ADVANCED BICEPS CONTROL

When you have learned to hump up the biceps while your arm is bent all the way, you have attained partial control. You are still in the state where your control is dependent on favorable arm positions. Complete mastery comes with the ability to flex the biceps at will, independent of position.

When the arm is fully bent (XLVI) the biceps bunches up naturally, as soon as you put tension on it. The next thing to do is to learn to make it project when the arm is half-bent; when the forearm and upper-arm are at right angles.

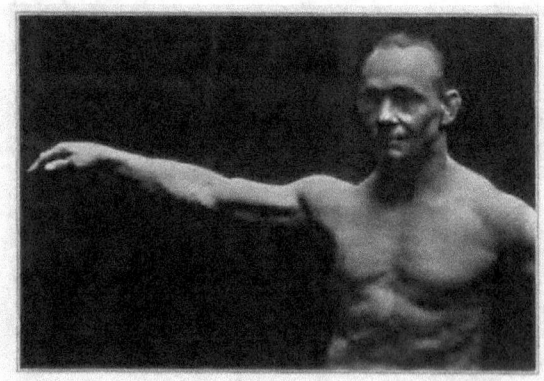

Figure XLVIII

In XLIX Arco's arm is a little past the right-angle position, yet the biceps rises in a high curve. Similarly you see pictures of athletes with their arm bent at right angles and a most surprising biceps display. Close to the forearm the upper-arm will be flat for an inch then curves in a sudden and abrupt semicircle. The biceps is not as big as when the arm is fully-bent: but its outline is different. It looks like the sun half-risen from a flat horizon. Mr. Mead is a wonder at this display. (See Figure LIII.) He did

100

something like in Figure 7 (October); only his arm was viewed from above. That picture greatly interested Arco. When at Scott's, I suggested that he try it. He made an attempt. Both of us forgot that Mead was leaning far over, so Arco only leaned over a little way. He tried several times and finally said "I have it. See! it is the thumb that does it." (We snapped Figure L.) When his arm was at right angles, the biceps did not rise high enough to suit him. His palm was away from the camera, he discovered that by turning the palm up and as much as possible towards the camera he could have the biceps project higher. Figure LI was another and less successful attempt. It was a new pose to Arco. You can see how intently he is watching his reflection in the mirror.

Every stunt like that, as it is mastered, makes one more degree of control: another subjection of the muscle to the will. It finally will become possible to display the biceps almost as much when the arm is halt bent, as when fully bent. Your will-power will make the muscle flex and swell no matter if the position is unfavorable.

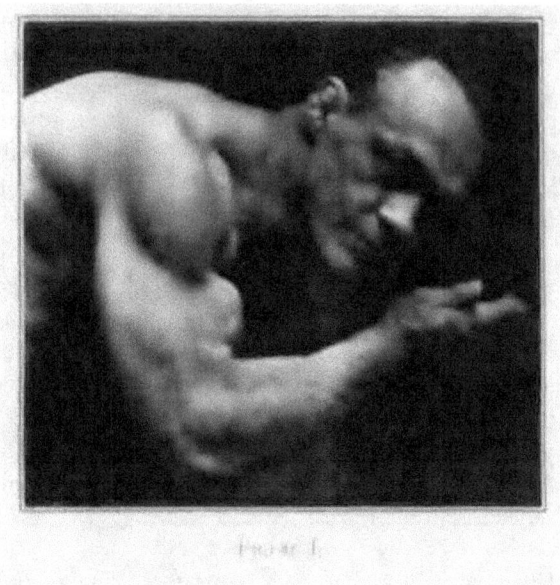

PLATE I

The hardest thing of all is to flex the biceps in the position of extension. XLVIII shows the biceps relaxed and perfectly smooth. In XLVII Arco has so strongly tensed the biceps that it looks sinewy and you can actually see the line of division between its two bellies. Otto says he does it by pushing strongly away with the hand, and by putting his thumb in the queer position shown. I can't tell you how to do it—can't explain it. It must be partly due to the amount of tension you put on the muscle. It isn't easy. We took four shots with the camera before we got it. The strain of concentration is reflected in the facial expression.

In getting control the foregoing is about all you need. Of course, there are other display stunts which can be suggested. An effective one is to face your audience; clasp your hands on top of your head and alternately flex and relax the biceps; first simultaneously; then right flexed, left relaxed; and then vice-versa rapidly. Putting the hands on the head lets you fully relax the biceps and make the subsequent contractions seem greater by comparison. When you bend the arm and hold the elbows up, there is bound to be some tension on the muscles which raise the arm; among which is the biceps. When you rest the hands on the crown of the head that support enables you to relax the muscles fully. That is one of the little things which are a help to beginners.

And by the way, you probably recognized Figure XLIX. It was used in the first circular announcing this magazine. Also it is part of the full-length picture of Arco which appeared on page 25 of "THE BROAD OF THE BACK". The arm was not so noticeable in that pose because it seemed to fit in so exactly with the width of the shoulders and the breadth of the back. When I wanted a picture of Arco's arm for the circular, I reproduced only that part of the photograph shown in XLIX. I centered the picture so that I practically compelled you to fix your gaze on the shoulder and upper-arm. Arco himself says that he thinks it is a wonderful view of his arm.

THE FORE-ARM

If you have ever studied pictures of well-muscled athletes, or if you have examined your physique by aid of a mirror, you must have noticed that it is hard to make the forearm and upper-arm look big at the same time.

When the upper-arm looks its biggest, the forearm is almost bound to look small, because you see it from the side (XLVI). On the contrary when you fix your arm so that the forearm seems very big, you are disappointed to note that the position is not the best for displaying the upper-arm. Perhaps the best combined effect is when the arm is bent half-way, as in XLIX, for then if you have the control, you can make the biceps stand up, can also harden the triceps to put the curve on the under side of the arm and make the forearm much wider than when the arm is fully bent.

What gives the breadth to the forearm in XLIX is the tightening of the supinator longus muscle. You will note on the picture that the lower edge of the forearm is one .almost straight line, starting near the base of the thumb and cutting into the upper arm just in front of where the biceps start. The lower tendon of that muscle is fastened to the lower end of the outer bone of the forearm. Its upper tendon is fastened to the upper-arm bone, a couple of inches above the elbow. As its name implies it is one of the muscles which rotate the forearm: but because it crosses the elbow-joint, it helps bend the arm at the elbow when it contracts.

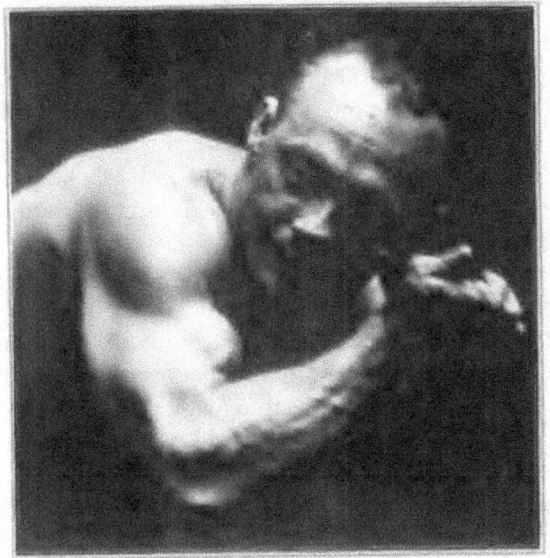

Figure LI

It is easy to get control of the supinator; in fact you may get it unconsciously while you are mastering the biceps. But it will not hurt to learn a little about its action. So stand facing your mirror; raise your arm to the side: bend it half-way at the elbow so that the forearm is perpendicular and palm of hand towards the mirror. Now tighten your biceps muscle. As the biceps hump up, you will see the supinator tighten. The forearm near the elbow will suddenly become almost fifty per cent thicker than before. The ability to make the supinator stand out increases very quickly.

To make the forearm look its very biggest, it is necessary to flex and control all of its muscles; ;is Arco is doing in LII. To duplicate the pose you have to limit your arm; tighten the supinator and then clench your fist and bend the wrist. As the palm of the hand is depressed then the hand itself must be rotated away from you, until the forearm is in what some call the "gooseneck position." You will never get those flexors on the inside of the forearm fully, merely bend the hand over. You have to rotate it as you bend. It enables you to contract the muscles so strongly that they cramp. And of course you have to do all that without once relaxing the supinator. You will be surprised how your forearm will actually build up by practicing this stunt. The gain in control is almost always accompanied with a gain in size and shape.

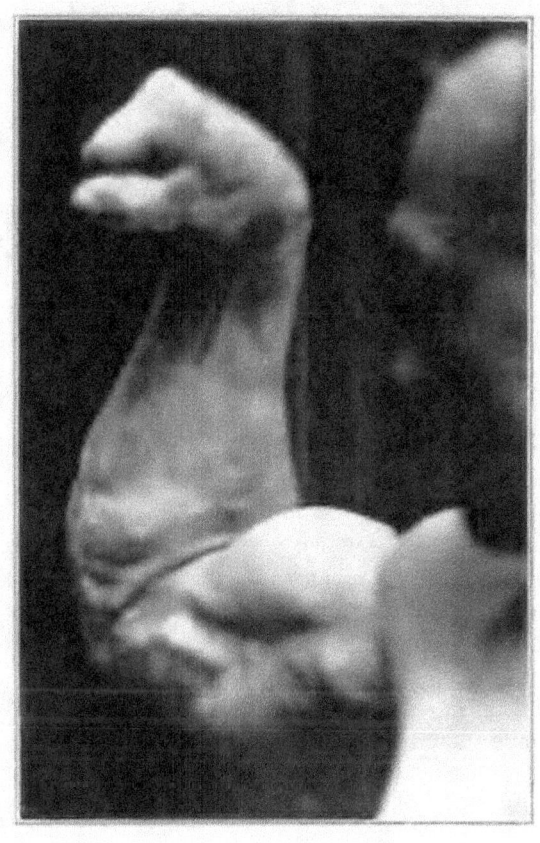

Figure 14

The foregoing reads more like an article on arm display than like a lesson in muscle-control. The answer is that muscle-tensing (muscular display) is based on muscle-control. That part about the forearm is an instance. You can't get the display unless you can make the muscles do what you want them to do.

When I first saw Sandow do it he gave the impression that he could alter the size and shape of his forearm at will. After doing the "gooseneck." he would open his hand, straighten the wrist and let all the forearm muscles go lax: and he would "gooseneck", relax, and repeat several times quickly. His forearm seemed to literally double in size while you were watching it.

This makes an ideal exercise providing you with alternate full contraction and full relaxation.

There is an advantage about this muscle-control which makes a great apnea to the non-athletes; especially to the man who wants exercise without the fatigue and soreness which follows violent work. You can practice muscle-control to the limit, and finish up fresh. And if you have spent half the time in alternating relaxation with contraction you never have any sore muscles.

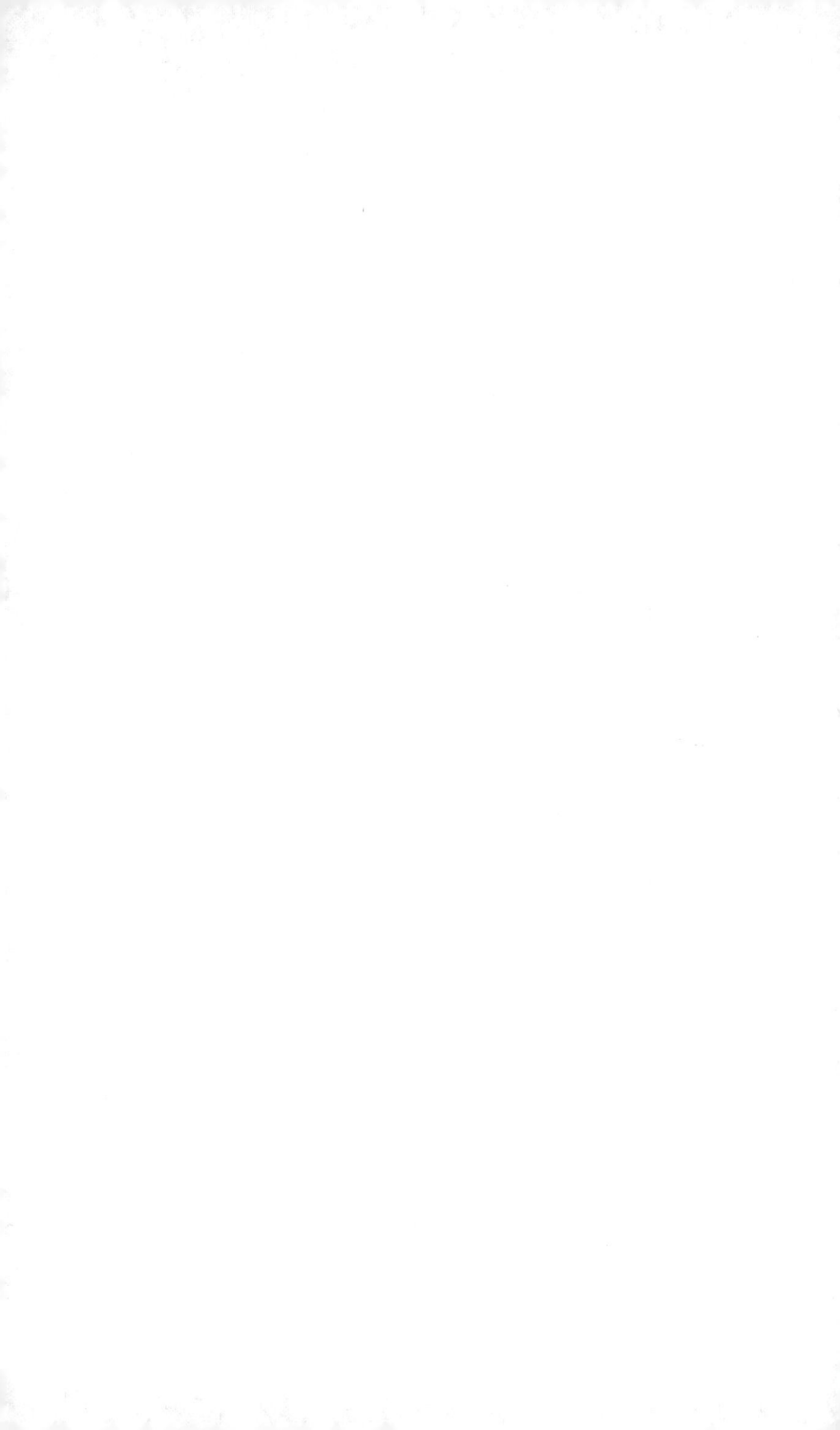